MY COLLECTION

The Road to Pleasure
Wine and Spirits

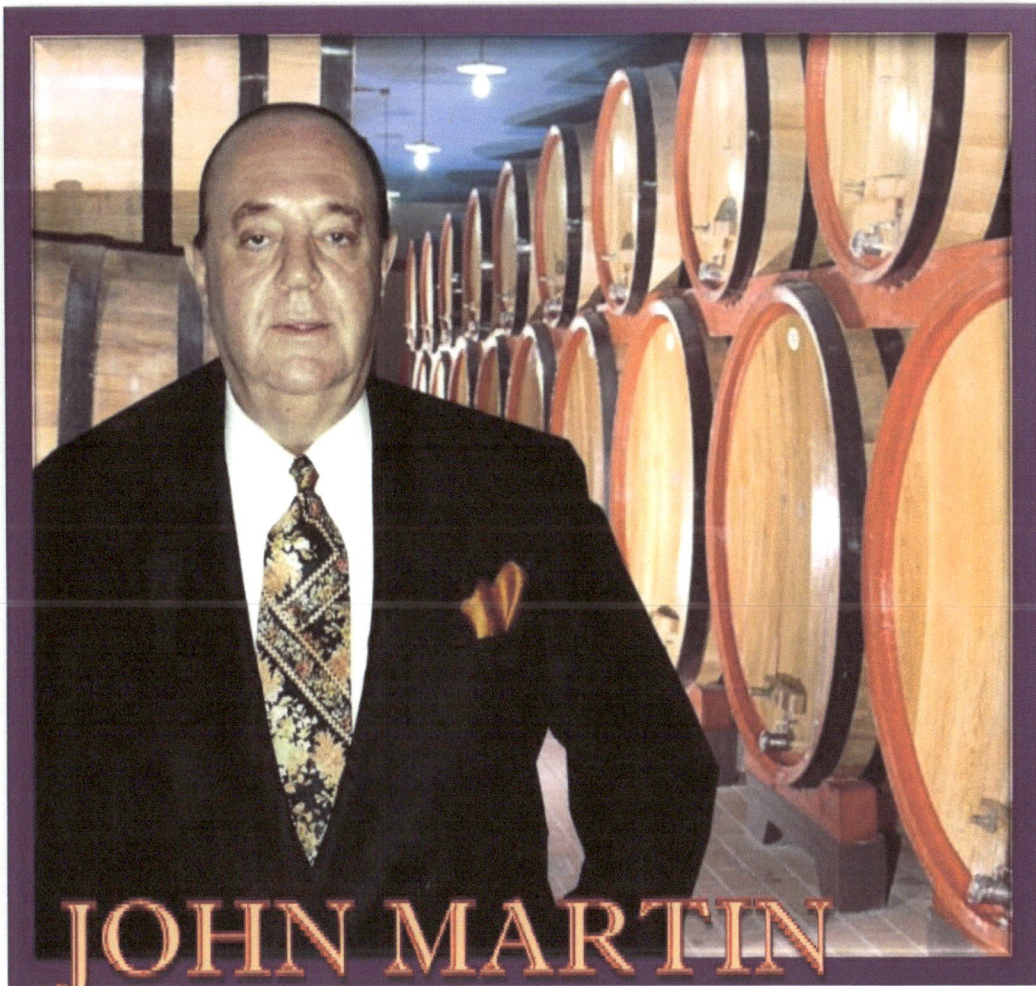

JOHN MARTIN

Thank you for your collaboration:
Carmen Roig Carvajal
Jason Whiting

ISBN-13: **978-9780900663**
ISBN-10: **9780900667**
My Collection. The Road to Pleasure.
Wine and Spirits
Authored by John Martin

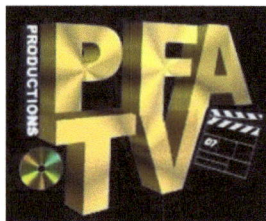

Florida. 305-244-6072

(Editorial Printed Fine Arts)

For my loving wife Vicky, a unique and great artist.

My inspiration to submerge in "The Road to Pleasure".

Yours, JOHN.

My Collection
"The Road to pleasure"

Prologue

The World of Wine and Spirits is a universe of physical and mental sensations, with great positive influence in everybody's life. The book you are about to read explains in full, in this great essay collection, its sources and elaboration. As John brilliantly explains, Wines in particular and Liquors in general, belong to a life with plenty of good health and happiness, unless an extreme abuse takes place causing dangerous diseases.

All Five Continents are producers of Wines and Spirits of different styles. There is no doubt that they are the best accompaniment with the daily food, banquets and all types of celebrations, due to its inspiring aromas and exotic flavors. All the reader's questions will be satisfied by the Author.

John Martin is already, for more than seventeen years, the brilliant Wine and Spirits Editor of **"Selecta"** Magazine and also a contributor for **"Casalife"** Magazine subsidiary of "Selecta", pouring his wise and accurate knowledge on the "The World of Wine and Spirits"

Open the door and go forward!

Michael Bulnes. President.
Revista Selecta

THE BEGINNING OF "THE ROAD OF PLEASURE"

Is an indisputable fact that the knowledge of Wines and Spirits, even in a general appearance, it is imperative owning it to function properly in the social life of today, both in the corporate events as in the social celebrations.

In summary, we must develop the ability to be able to choose the wines and spirits concordant with menus for lunches, brunches, cocktail parties, family meals, and evenings of exotic classic style and dinners of Grand Gala. Nor should we forget the importance of being able to respond appropriately to questions of our guests or colleagues of events. This will be the task!

It is noteworthy as the Wine and Spirits capture our five senses: "The View" allows us to appreciate the Color, anticipating the purity of the method. "The Smell" provides the aroma and tells us if the product is finished and ready to taste. "The Taste" reaffirms the impression of the smell at the beginning, and then creates a round movement in the mouth, reveals to us the Bouquet, permeating the nasal area, sending a mandate to the brain based on the comparison with the subconscious, where are stored all the prints prior to the type of wine or spirit tasted. "The Touch", perhaps unnoticed, resides in the lightness, finesse and transparency of the glass that carries the nectar and to "The Ear" establishing the "Chin-Chin", a gesture of love and friendship in fine Bacarract.

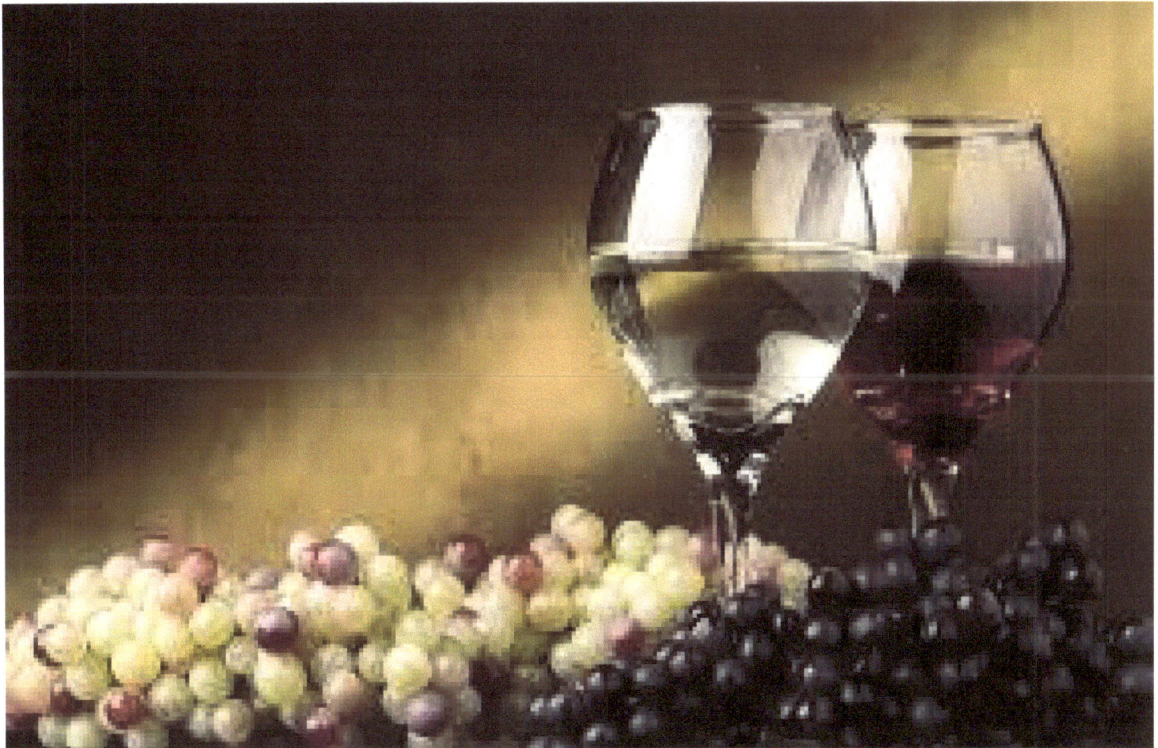

THE ROTHSCHILD

The most notorious financial conglomerate recognized worldwide within the wine industry.

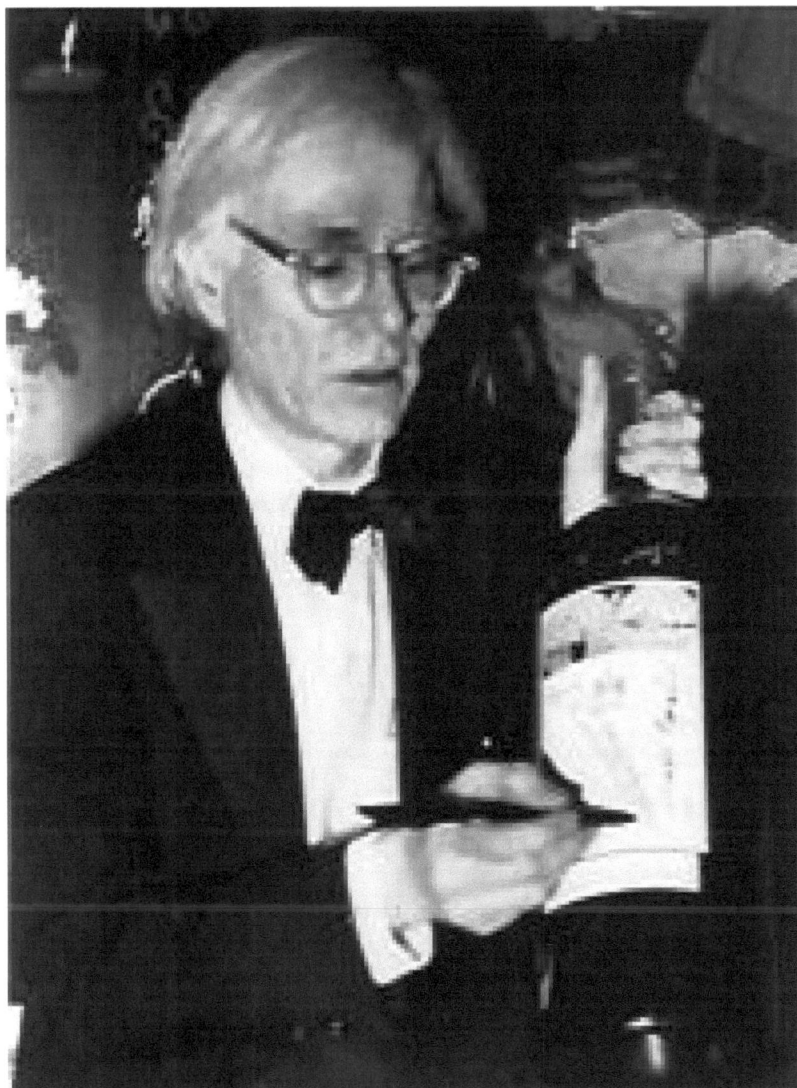

In 1743, in the city of Frankfurt, saw the light for the first time Mayer Anselm Rothschild, founder of a dynasty universally recognized by the vast economic, political, and social contribution to the history of many countries throughout the world.

The financial and social success of the House of Rothschild (Red Shield in Spanish) is due to a simple principle: the close family harmony. From the Napoleonic Wars of the one thousand eight hundred, period of eminence historic to the Dynasty, until the Wall Street of today, the Rothschild have been an example of economic socio-political vision.

Mayer and his five sons, Anselm, Solomon, Nathaniel (financial whiz of the family) Karl and James were commissioned to solidify its influence in the world bank established in Frankfurt, Vienna, London, Naples and Paris respectively. The Crown of Austria, forming part of the European aristocracy, appointed all of them Barons.

Meteriocally their investments were extended beyond the banking covering various businesses, among them agriculture. In 1868 Baron James de Rothschild, a great lover of wine, purchased the 100 hectares of vineyard more famous in the world. Château Lafite in Pauillac. James had his eyes on Lafite since 1855, the year in which this wine without torque was proclaimed the "premier des premiers "Grand Cru", Medoc. With his purchase of Lafite de Rothschild he came through the big door leading the Wine aristocracy.

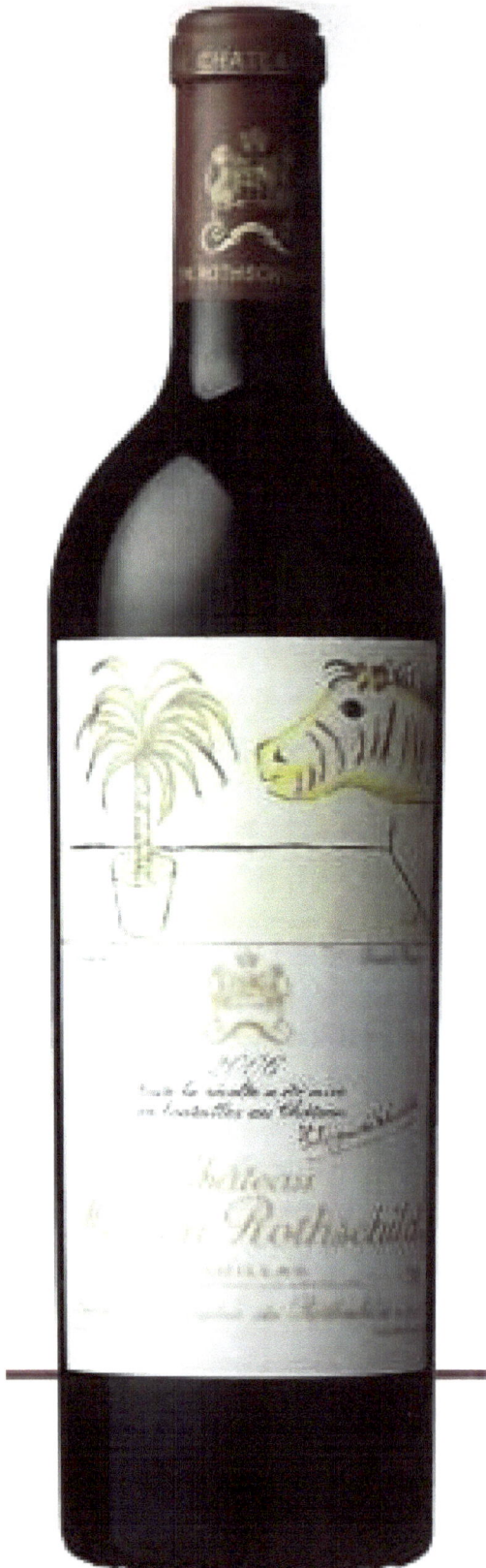

Domain Lafite Rothschild: 100 years before this happened, the Cardinal Richelieu, Prime Minister of Louis XV, consulted with their physician on the state of their health due to a long journey that they were going to undertake. The doctor prescribed the wine of Château Lafite as the best and most enjoyable of the tonics. On their return, Louis XV told Richelieu that his appearance was that of a man 25 years younger, to what the Cardinal replied: *"Your Majesty knows that I have found the famous Fountain of Youth. I have discovered that the wine of Château Lafite is friendly generous, delicious and comparable to the Ambrosia of the gods of the Olympo".* As a result, the king declared the wine as the official of Versailles, with the approval of Madame de Pompadour and Madame du Barry. The most benefited from this was the owner of the vineyard, Alexandre de Segur, known by the nickname of *"the Prince of the Vineyards".*

In the present Château Lafite Rothschild, thanks to the quality of the "terroir" planted with the classical strains of Médoc, Cabernet Sauvignon (70 %), Merlot (25 %), Cabernet Franc (3 %) and Petit Verdot (2 %), continues to be the wine most coveted of the world. A product scented, bright and chivalrous with property of long aging.

The Domain, now led by Baron Eric de Rothschild, produces and also controls a selection of elegant wines of high quality:

Carruades of Lafite and Château Duhart-Milon (Pauillac), Château Peyre-Lebade (Haut-Medoc), Château L'évangile (Pomerol), Château Portillo (Sauternes), Quinta do Carmo (Alentejo Portuguese), The Basques (Chile) Catena (Argentina), Echelon (California Coast), Acacia (Napa in California), Canoe Ridge (Washington State), Ruppert - Rothschild (South Africa) and Tyrrell's (Australia).

In the business of wine today the Rothschild have won four of the five continents. Mouton Rothschild: The original property called Brane Mouton in the commune of Pauillac, 30 miles northwest of Bordeaux, was acquired in 1853 by Baron Nathaniel de Rothschild, director of the English branch of the family business, and renamed it Mouton Rothschild combining two wonders, the fruitful land of the vineyards of Medoc and the spirit of a family famous for its success and sophistication. However there was a vigorous intervention on the part of its members until 1922 in which a young man of 20 years, great grandson of Nathaniel, enamored of his social position and its vineyards, took in his hands the future of Mouton. It was Philippe de Rothschild.

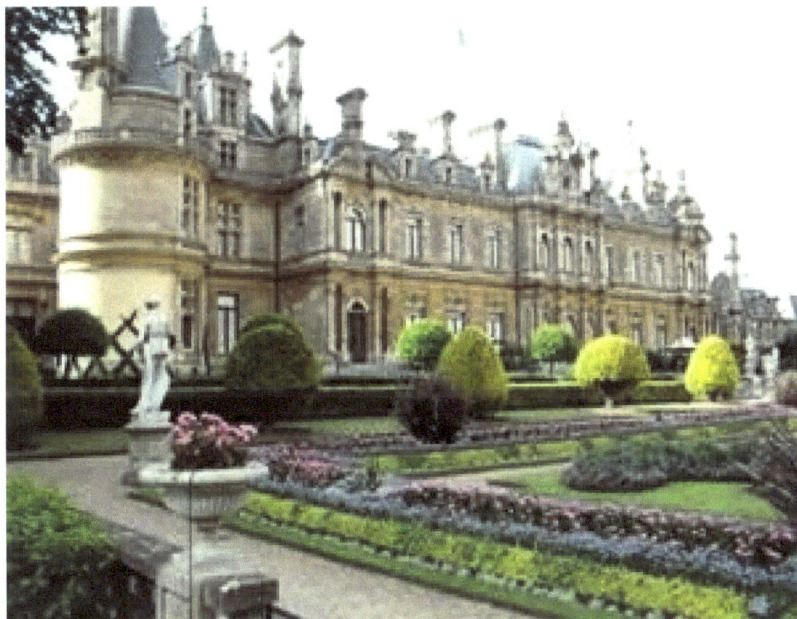

Contrary to the traditionalism of Lafite, Philippe appears as an innovator with its Mouton. As a young visionary he became in a short time a master of production and dissemination. Their ideas are revolutionizing the market inventing the bottling in the same Château, system that was since then adopted by the majority of the wineries of renown, giving their wines an air of family prestige.

Philippe boldly assembled several types of wines creating the first mark of name Bordeaux, Mouton Cadet. He also transformed the labelling by resorting to the great artists of his time to illustrate those of its unsurpassed Château Mouton Rothschild.

He was the first European winegrower that, in partnership with Robert Mondavi, develops in the heart of the Napa Valley the best wine of America, Opus One, father of the Meritage Californian. Until his death in 1988 always followed the same rule, an eye on the tradition and another in the innovation. A few years before his death, the daughter of Baron Philippe de Rothschild, Phillipine, actress in the French Comedy, abandons her scenarios to join his father and help him in his crusade.

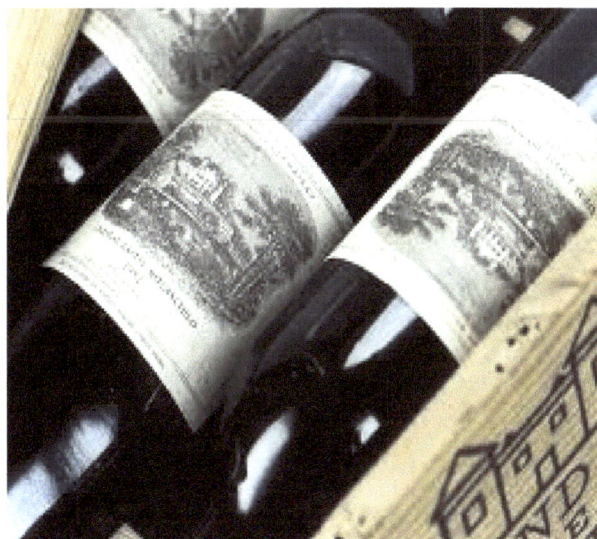

Under the spirit of support of the Baron, Baroness Philippine currently works in close collaboration with the Directorate General of Mouton to maintain, modernize and develop the family business.

Accompanying the "Premier Cru Classé" Château Mouton Rothschild (Pauillac), the company of Baron Phillipe offers us:

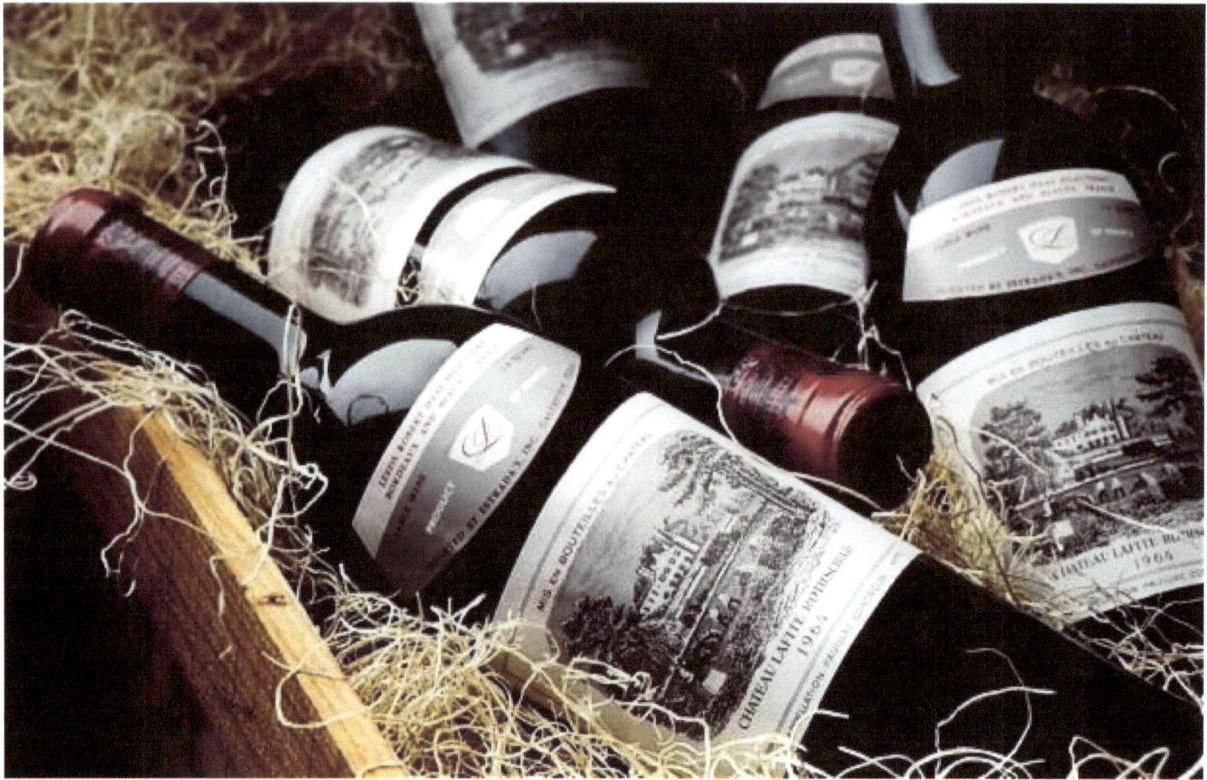

Château d'Armailhac
Château Clerc Milon
Le Petit Mouton (all of Pauillac)
Aile d'Argent (Bordeaux)
Château Coutet and Chartreuse Coutet (Sauternes-Barsac)
Vin Sec Château Coutet (serious)
Mouton Cadet Reserve (Medoc)
Mouton Cadet (Bordeaux)
Varietals of Cabernet Sauvignon
Merlot, Chardonnay and Sauvignon Blanc (all of the country of Oc)
Opus One (California)
Red Shield (Chile) and certain selections limited wine bordaleses.

"My only ambition is to make the best wines in the world".
Baron Phillipe de Rothschild.

LA RIOJA AND RIBERA DEL DUERO

The most illustrious Denominations of Origin of Spanish Wine.

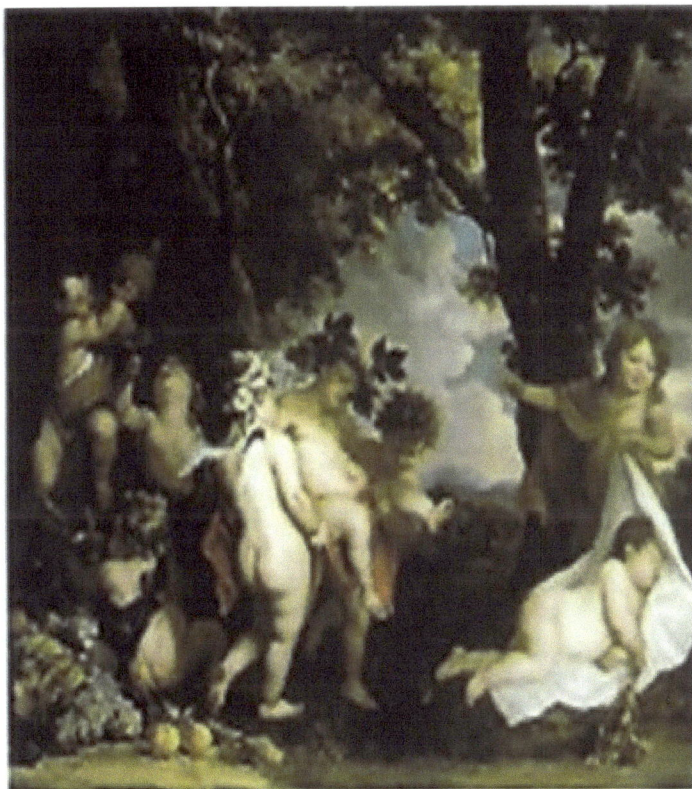

With the exception of certain wineries individually established in different areas of the Iberian Peninsula, the domain of La Rioja, until the 1980s was the source of domestic production and international distribution of the most noble wines of Spain.

From the beginning of the 1990s, this region, a pioneer in the art of making wine had to face the competition of the increasing production of the New Spanish wine, from a large number of different wine-growing areas. This phenomenon was highly positive for **La Rioja**, which opened the door to creativity and virtuosity of their teacher winemakers, currently featuring in the market the more advanced methods of cultivation and wine production. A wide variety of new grapes, apart from the traditional Tempranillo, allowed blends of unique character.

In 1982 was officially established the Ribera del Duero, seated in the heart of Castilla becoming the most formidable competitor of La Rioja. Their wines more notable, red wines in its majority, suffer from a color exceptionally dark, are superbly fruity, with a robust body and are aged in American or French oak. The most prominent grape is the Tinta del País or Tinta Fina, equivalent to the Tempranillo variety.

The following is an informative example of the other of these regions, also the pride of the Spanish wine industry:

Prado Rey – Real Sitio de Ventosilla (Ribera del Duero): Their apparent existence covers a long chapter in the history of Spain.

In 1503 Isabel La Católica acquired this monumental venue on behalf of the Crown of Castile with the purpose to provide the Court with a place of recreation, leisure and abundance of big game.
The Bodegas Prado Rey, rest between rugged hills and rich vineyards that grow in a deep and sandy soil, typical of the Ribera del Duero. Don Javier Cremades, one of the most illustrious businessman of Spain, owner of Ventosilla, says: *"In our wines are being met the expectations of their consumers, all lovers of culture known as the world of wine"*.

We recommend: **Crianza** and **Reserva**. Aged for a minimum of 7 years.

Elite - The jewel of the collection. All the Prado King are recommended with roasts, game, red meats and most of the modern Iberian Kitchen dishes.

Dinastía Vivanco - La Rioja Alta. Those who throughout the ages have forged the history of Wine have been characters that, in most cases, have been trained in agricultural and geological techniques. This group know the exact methods to reach the summit of the production of the elixir, encouraging the passionate love of the same. But how do those who have preserved with fervour tangible signs of the eternal culture wine? Don Pedro Vivanco, the current patriarch of the fourth generation of winemakers of La Rioja, who, with his Foundation erected the Wine Museum, unique in the world to host a rich collection of old tools, works of art and archaic documents related exclusively to the world of wine. Its 300 hectares of vineyards lie at the foot of the Sierra de Cantabria in La Rioja Alta on the banks of the Ebro river. Apart from the Dinastia Vivanco wines, the family owns several other wineries in La Rioja, including Carlos Serres, Castillo de Clavijo and other breeders of La Rioja.

Must try: **Crianza 2001** (100% Tempranillo:Bright and deep purple color. Intense aroma of ripe fruit, vanilla and spices. Toasted *bouquet* with a lingering and elegant finish. **Reserve 1998** (90% Tempranillo, 10% Graciano): Cherry red color garrnets with bright and clean traits. Great harmony of noble tannins. Complex and elegant with a long finish.

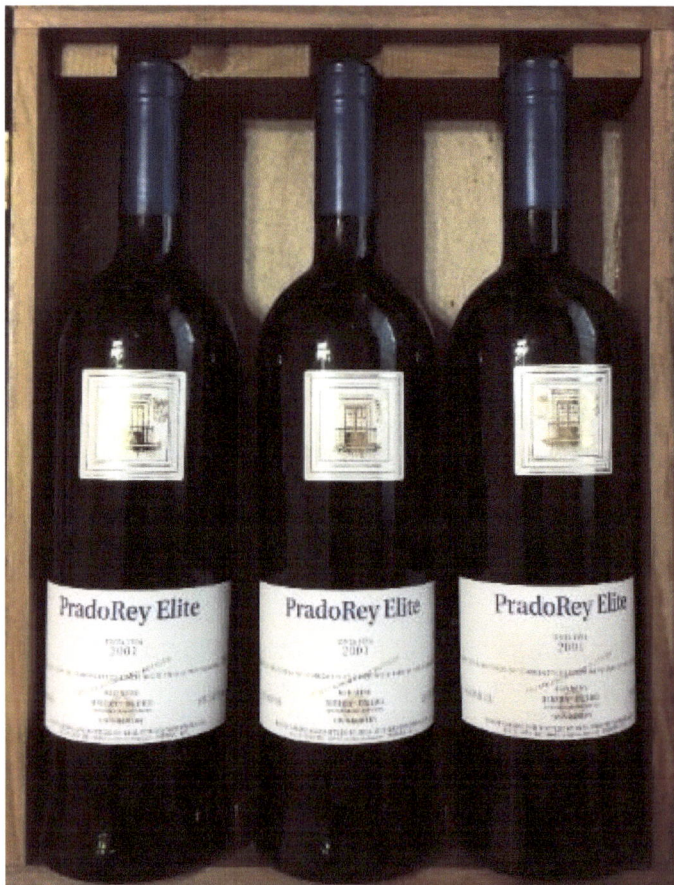

All wines with great style, representative of their land and with a great intrinsic value.

WINE AND INTERNATIONAL POLITICS

France returns to our market with more force and aggressiveness than ever

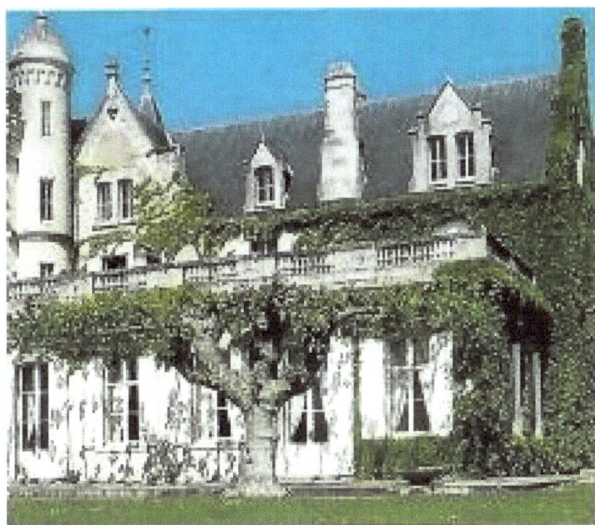

Universal History shows us since ancient times, the actual existence of the commercial isolation as a powerful weapon in war times and ideological or diplomatic conflicts: If the country "A", a great political influence and economic power, differs with the country "B", industrious and liberal, on an argument of a political nature, the country "A", using an ardent Public Relations campaign, sets in motion a commercial blockade that carries a considerable loss to the country "B".

The most recent example we has been witnessed during the past three years: Country "A", the United States and France, the locked country "B", faces a dismal drop in exports of their products in the American market. In particular the Wine. It is general knowledge the historic tradition and unrivalled quality of French wines, so I am inclined to think that the real losers are the consumers, which, I can assure without any doubt, they prefer a Château Lafite to political slogans. This feeling has been reflected in the successful recurrence of French wine in America, already distant of bickering inconsequential rumors. Curious Note: The sale of Champagne is rapidly rising.

Now, back to normalcy, I am going to have the pleasure of referring to our readers the merits of a Bordeaux wine that has been considered, for more than 300 years, as a member of the top French Wine: the "Grand Cru Classé **Château Lascombes**", designation Margaux. The foundation of the vineyard in 1625, is due to the Chevalier Antoine Lascombes. The classification of Grand Cru Classé was conferred in 1855, until, almost a century later in 1952. The property was acquired by Alexis Lichine one of the most prestigious authorities in the Wine industry. The vineyards and wineries have been completely renovated and restructured causing admiration among the members of the Wine industry. At present, the owners of **Château Lascombes** and their second wine **Chevalier de Lascombes**, constitute a substantial private financial group of shareholders, led by Sebastien Bazin, main investor of the company who has an illustrious professional team. Dominique Befve, its Director General, was an integral part of the **Châteaux Lafite Rothschild** and **Duhart-Milon**, as well as Director of the wineries of the **Château L'évangile**, Pomerol. All of the aforementioned modern companies, are technically advanced models of the new style of the Médoc wines, presented recently in the market their first vintages. **Château Lascombes**, Margaux, 2001: Deep blackberry color. Aroma of red fruits, elegantly linked with the oak in explosive *bouquet* with a long slightly chocolate final. **Château Lascombes**, Margaux, 2002: Intense color that reveals the presence of strawberries of the forest and touches of roasted coffee. One can appreciate a slight touch of pepper and subtle tannins. Powerful and distinguished yielding a great potential for long aging. **Chevalier de Lascombes** 2001: a wine to drink young, enjoying its softness and new style.

This great wine returned to stay. Cheers!

HEIGHTENING THE PRESENCE OF THE WINE INSIDE AND OUT OF THE BOTTLE

Suggestions dictated by the art of presenting and of tasting the Good Wine

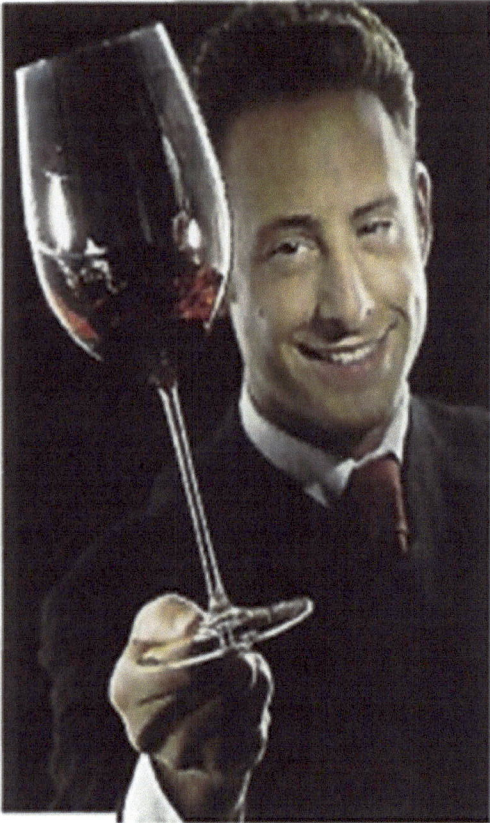

The Glass: Since the human race integrated to the anthropological history of our planet, the need to consume the basic fluids to maintain the perpetuity of its species created the need to invent functional receptacles that were suitable to contain the liquids to be consumed From an immemorial period, a series of gadgetry rescued from History appeared namely the *amphorae* and the glasses of different designs.

The clay and the wood were the raw material preferred for its power of isolation of the environment assuring its preservation until the crystal did its appearance.

Glasses dating of the year 2200 BC were in decimated areas of Persia and Babylonia, but what does not leave any doubt is the crystal gadgetry found in Egypt during the reign of the Pharaoh Amenhotep II (1448 BC) arising hence from now on the continued manufacture of receptacles and crystal glasses. Considering the Middle East the documented cradle of the Wine, the use of this style of solid and profusely decorated receptacles, was adopted in Egypt and later in Greece and Rome like the ideal way of consumption.

Claus Riedel, in the middle of 1600s opened the doors of its factory of glasses, vases and artistic crystal objects in Bohemia, presently belonging to the Czech Republic.

Nowadays, eleven generations later, Maximilian Riedle, CEO of Riedel Crystal, carries the banner of the family, presenting to the world the most finished and varied collection of glasses of Wine of the thinnest crystal and unique manufacture. Riedle was the first one in the industry that discovered the importance of the

El estilo Art Deco no podía faltar. Indicado para licores finos

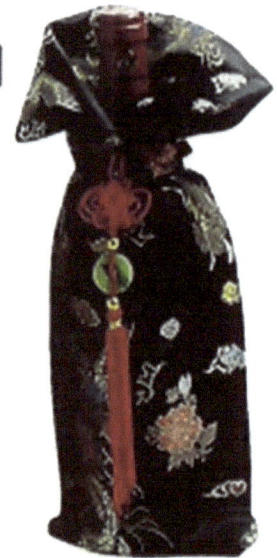

Colección de rasgos orientales en satén y seda

glass design for the specific tasting of every wine. Certain geometric principles and handmade blown, coiling lightly the rims of the glass, heightens the aroma and the bouquet to the maximum. They make different style lines for its selection.

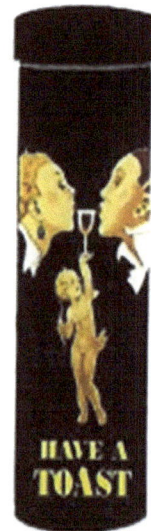

Giving away a bottle of Wine or Liquor with style and social awareness: Recently a group of friends graduated in Business Administration in Berkeley University, decided to convince the consumers that the wrapping paper bags were not worth carrying wines or class spirits, especially when having these presented as a gift of personal affection. With this philosophy, True Fabrications marketed a variety of more than 150 designs of bags for wine and liquor for gift and transportation, which included *papier maché* boxes with pressed wild flowers of the Himalayas, bags of hemp woven by hand, decorated on any color and stamped bundles of satinwood and silk. It should noted that all models need to be properly reusables. In the brief time of successful operations, the company has penetrated in over 3,000 establishments offering its products across North America and they can be Found in 49 of our 50 states (seemingly it is not drunk very much in Utah).

This year's expansions are projected to Canada and England. It is a presentation of big class and style. For its expediency all the models are reusables. For convenience, contact True Fabrications Internet route: www.truefabric.com.

Farewell to "brown bags" !!!

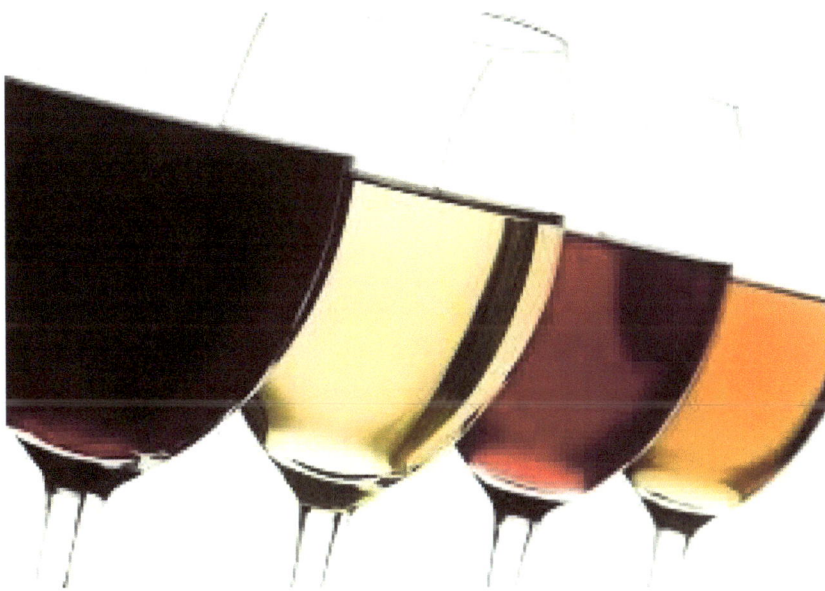

WHISKY, THE "WATER OF LIFE" IN SCOTLAND

Enjoyed by more than five hundred years ago is today the most popular of the planet

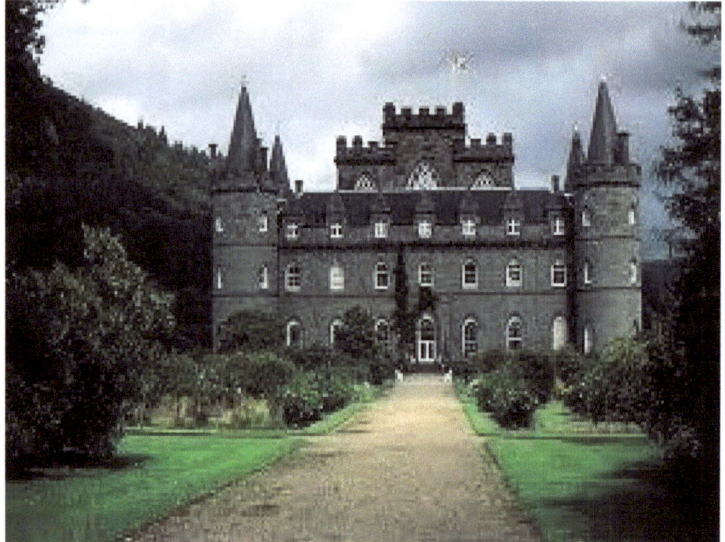

During the beginning of the tenth century the Arabic Alchemist Al-Bukassen revealed in his writings the distillation process, which travelled toward the four cardinal points. Initially conceived for medicinal and healing purposes due to the emergence of alcohol, its initial purpose was changed committing this process for drinking consumption with altogether different purposes.

At present, distillation offers to the world a multitude of products that are part of the social structure of humanity. These "elixirs" spread throughout Western Europe since the early 1400s baptized *Aqua Vitae* in Latin, equivalent to *Water of Life* in English.

In the highlands of Great Britain, the tribe of the Scotts of prehistoric background , is believed to have emigrated from Ireland, created their own distillation process: the *uisgebeatha*, literal translation of Aqua Vitae to the Celtic language. Over time, its name was changed to the anglicism **Whisky** in Scotland and **Whiskey** in Ireland and the United States.

Scotland, without a doubt, is the cradle of the distillate, a paradoxical drink made with meager and humble ingredients infinitely varied and often of incredible complexity. Wise combination of grains crowned by malted barley pearl is essential. The whisky of "Single Malt" has an unmatched quality. Always processed in copper stills, linked to water purity without equal and leaving it to sit in a cask of white oak, opening doors to an unlimited aging. Result, a creamy spirit that must be tasted blended with a touch of water only. The Scottish style!.

Domestic distilleries reigned since immemorial time. It was impossible not to find in humble homes, castles of nobility, canteens of travellers or in the backpack of the Guerrero in the presence of the whisky home. Hard, rough and exaggeratedly smoked. Commercial distillation was not regulated until 1814 in which the government imposed a tax on the production and sale of whisky. A new era began. Currently more than 100 distilleries compete for the excellence of the National Treasury.

The example of tradition and highest quality brings a whisky from Strathisla, number one in sales volume in the world: The Chivas Regal, product of the most celebrated mixtures of Scottish malts combined with fine and soft specially selected whiskies was the dream of its founders. The Chivas Brothers became a reality. In the whisky world market, Chivas 12 Year Old and Chivas 18 Year Old are the firstborn of the family. Within the category of whiskies long vintage Chivas Brothers offers us Royal Salute 21 & 51 Year Old.

Chivas 12, as it is called in the scope complex flavors, boasts a radiant amber and presents a master mix of single Scottish malts. Apple, honey, vanilla and hazelnut wrapped in an infusion of wild herbs are the more distinctive aromas of this wonderful scotch whisky nosing for 12 years in barrels of American white oak.

Join the family!

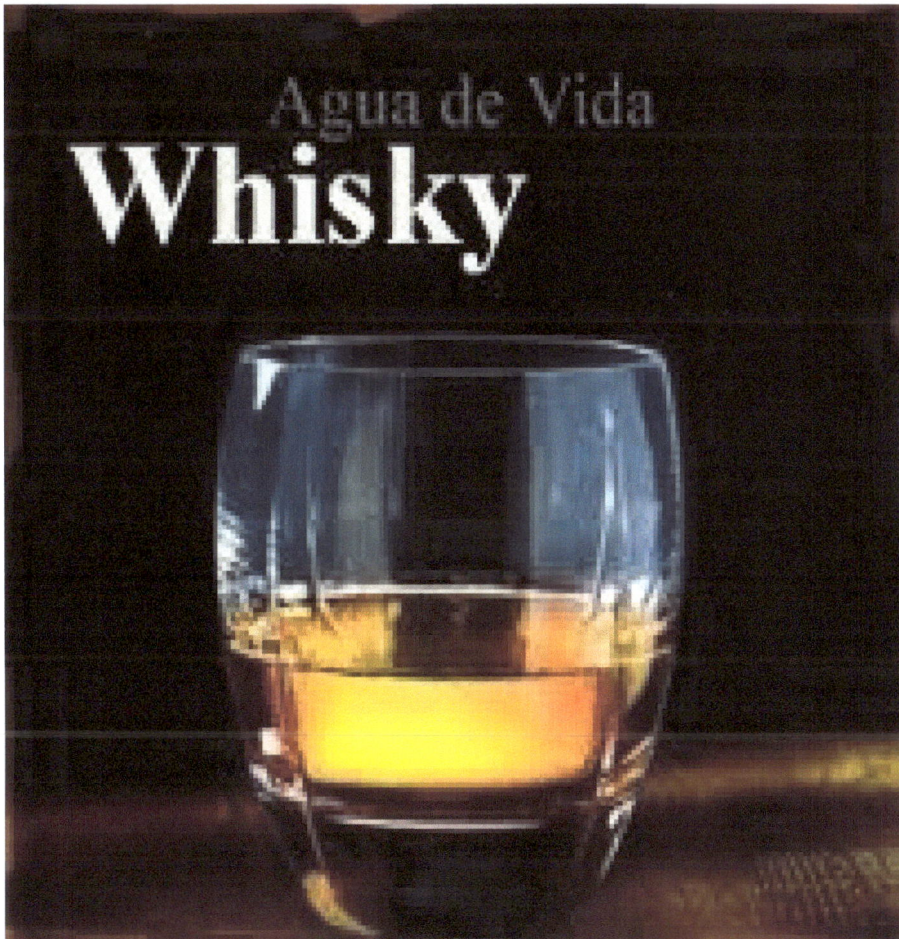

WINE AND "TAPAS": THE ART OF EATING STANDING

The delicious energy that illuminates the night of the successful Tapas Bar throughout Spain

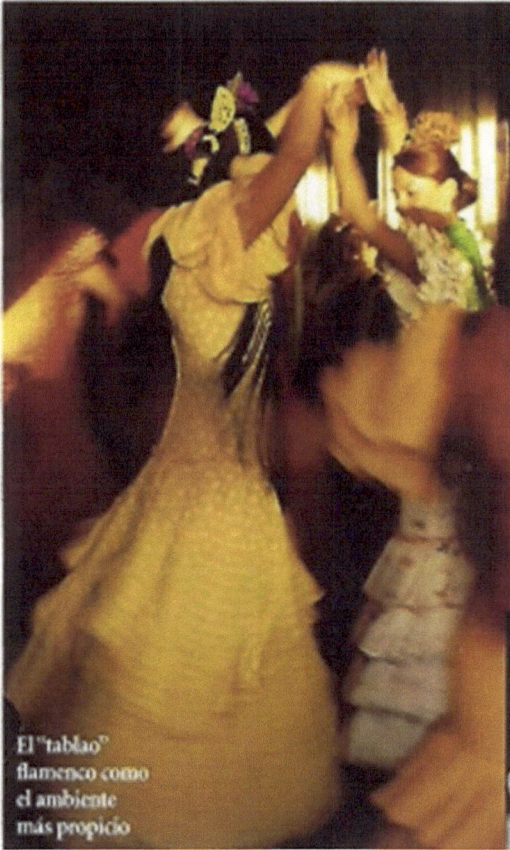

El "tablao" flamenco como el ambiente más propicio

It is impossible to explain why the majority of the events most brilliant and bright of the history of gastronomy have arisen by accident, error, or chance. However, it is a fact supported by a multitude of examples. There is more than 450 years of history coming from the Royal Crown of Philip II of the Hapsburg Dynasty. He established an eclectic reign of more than 70 years, which allowed him to pass by a multitude of psychological stages in his long existence as a Monarch. One of his customs for many years was walking often incognito into *colmados* and *tavernas* of Madrid without any escort, only in the company of his personal secretary Don Antonio Perez. Their raids had a dual purpose, enjoy an authentic and vibrant spirit folk sipping the wine of Castilla and pay attention with caution to the comments made around, allowing them to gauge the level of loyalty of the Spanish people. One of those so many nights, the King lifted his glass of wine to toast with Don Antonio. " By accident, error, or chance ", a dead fly floated on the surface of the King's Valdepeñas wine. Grossed out, the Monarch urged his secretary to leave the place immediately.

In brief, a Royal Decree ordered that glasses of wine were served throughout Spain using a "cover" for reasons of hygiene. The owners of the establishments did not like the idea, but obeyed without question. In order to comply with the Royal Decree, the merchants cut and varnished wooden circles, but the consumer considered it as an oddity of the King. Shortly after came the creative solution of the entrepreneurs: slices of ham, sausages, or any other delicacy presented in small portions, adorned the *"tapas"* of the wine giving way to 'THE FIRST COVER' in history, which was instituted until today, being treated as a way of eating and *"copear"* with a dynamic style, casual and festive.

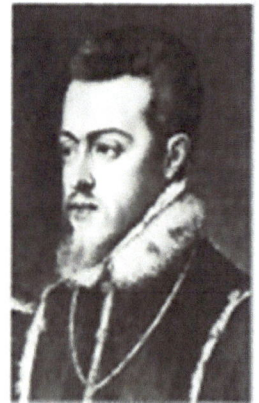

As a result wines with sensual *bouquet* emerged. In the world market. .

Never would have Felipe II imagined that his Royal Decree of the wooden covers were going to be such a success in the Wine World of today.

Thanks to a wine loving King!

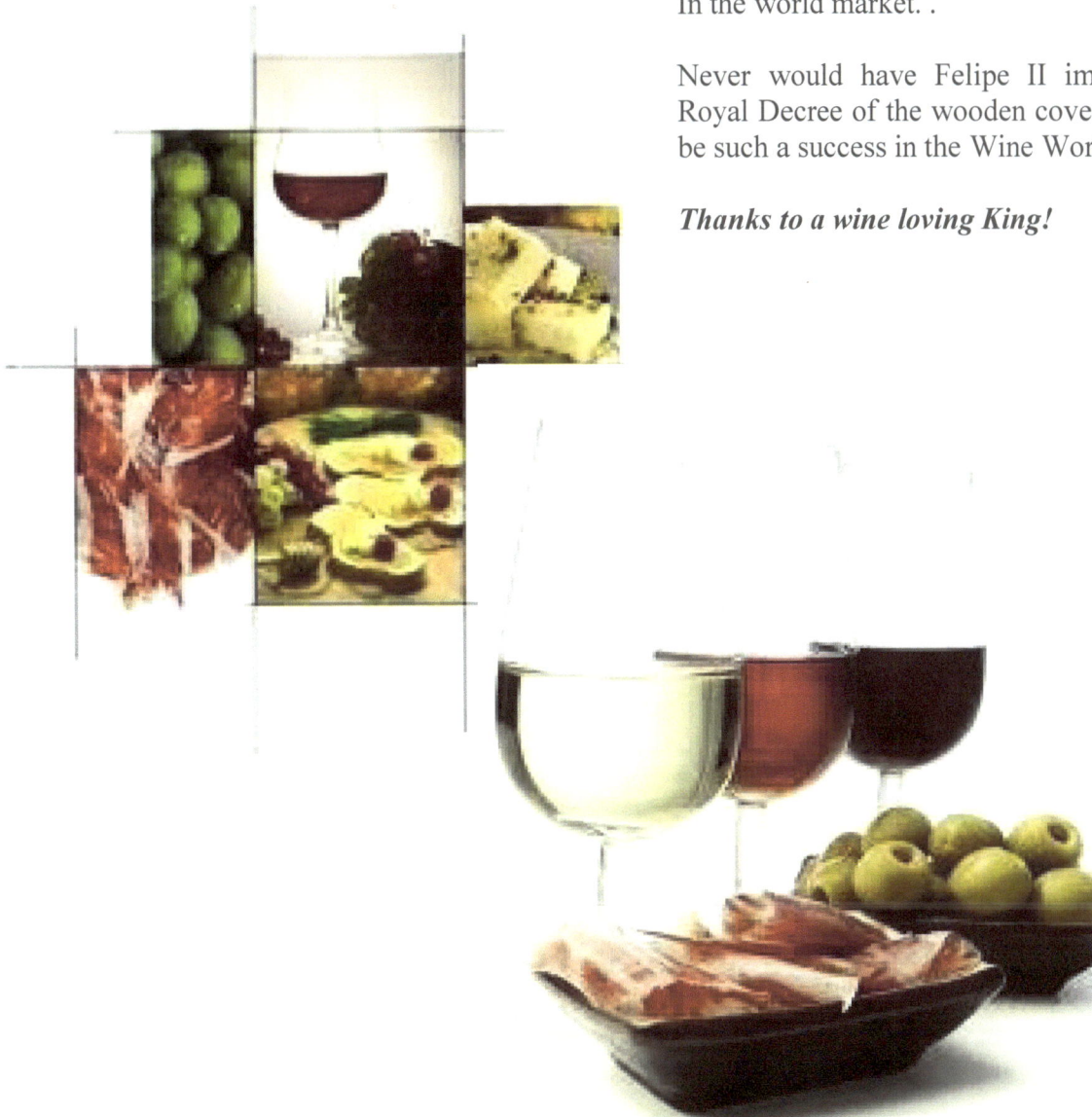

THE WINES OF "CALIENTE FORNALLA"

One of the most fertile regions of the world, known as California

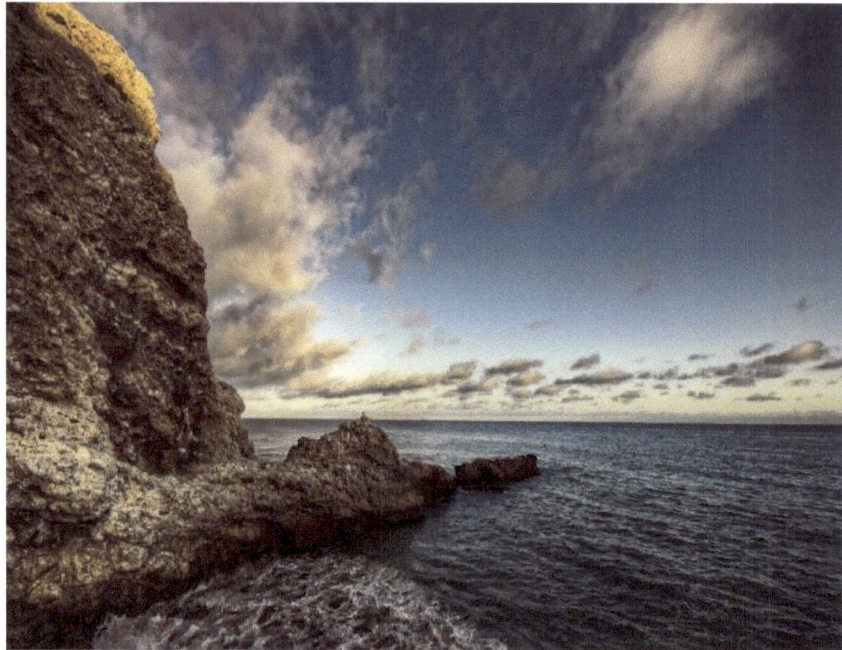

Occupying a coastal strip of the Pacific Ocean from more than 1.250 miles in length to the southwestern United States is California, the state of increased population and the second in extension after Texas. Its eastern boundary, dominated by the Sierra Nevada and the wilderness of Mohave, constitutes an inhospitable area due to the searing heat and its persistent dryness. Between these limits of opposite climatic characteristics one can fined the Central Valley, a corridor of 50 miles wide considered as one of the most fertile regions of the world. In particular, this región, is excelent for the cultivation and vinification of the vine. Due to this type of climate, the Spanish conquistadors baptised these lands, in old spanish, "Caliente Fornalla" or "hot oven".

There is still the notion that the California wine remains something "new", an attempt to emulate the sophisticated European wines. Nothing could be further from the truth. At the end of the nineteenth century their wines had been awarded with top honors in international competitions in Europe, as well as their agricultural products and livestock. A large immigration of producers and merchant including the prestigious Prussian winemaker Charles Krug emerged at the beginning of the 1900s looking to settle in the areas of Napa, Sonoma, Mendocino and sorrounding regions with a single intention: "Use your experience in the art of winemaking", opening the door for what today is the most extensive and lucrative market in the world. Thus were born some of today's most fabled winemaking companies of California. Unfortunately in 1919, due to the moral desires and puritan political circles in the country, the Constitution was amended by instituting the "prohibition" to the production, sale and use of alcohol. A stab in the heart of the wine.

In 1933, the United States voted to approve amendment 23, defeating the reign of the hypocrisy. This was the expected time for entrepreneurs to develop the rule of Californian wine.

Ernest and Julio Gallo, children of Italian immigrants founded their wineries in the Sonoma Valley in the same year that the prohibition was abolished. They had to get capital to start their activities that required the production of 185.000 gallons of sweet wines to be packaged and sold to the popular market. Today the bodegas E. & J. Gallo have an annual production of roughly 720 million bottles of wine of different characters. In 1943, Robert Mondavi, the monarch of the Cabernet Sauvignon, acquired the fabulous winery of Charles Krug.

This gave him the opportunity to improve his Cabernet and develop new european style vinification such as Chenin Blanc and Smoke Blanc. In 1979, associated with Baron Phillipe de Rothschild, presented to the world Opus One, the father of the Californian Meritage dinasty.

Currently, 90% of the wine produced in the United States comes from California, with New York, being the main consumer of the product. 65% of wines sold in hotels, restaurants and liquor stores in America are from California companies. Innumerable awards and honorific mentions have been granted to California wines in international exhibitions and its exportation grows amazingly. The wine barrels of more prestige in Europe have tackled associations in California taking refuge in its ideal climatological characteristics and in the quality of the American oak for aging in casks.

California invented and imposed in the world market production, wines made from a single type of grape, forcing the rest of the global wineries to mimic this process. The most acclaimed are Chardonnay, Sauvignon Blanc, Smoke Blanc, Pinot Gris, Chenin Blanc, Merlot, Syrah, Cabernet Sauvignon, Pinot Noir and Zinfandell. Sparkling wines are of great quality and one would be happy to recommend any of the incomparable "J", sparkling Californian par excellence.

Viva Californial!

THE ABSINTHE: THE "GREEN FAIRY" OF THE SPIRITS

Since the time of Hippocrates and Galeno until Hemingway and Picasso, this powerful and controversial beverage influenced the world of Medicine, Literature, Politics and the Arts

In the history of western culture never existed an elixir which led the glorious and brightest minds than the *Artemissia Absinthium*. The origin of the distillate known as Absenta in Spanish, conventionally known as Absente, in French and Absinthe in the English language. These semantic terms are universally used referring to this spirit.

This wild plant, discovered in the Val de Travers in the Swiss Jura is documented for the first time during the second century in the Herbarius treaty of the great philosopher Apuleius and mentioned and used by Hippocrates, the father of medicine, and the illustrious physician Galeno for the cure of various neurological and digestive deseases. In 1597, John Gerard, an eminent british herbalist, baptized our protagonist as Wormwood, recommended in his treaty Herball to neutralize the intestinal parasites. Later, in the seventeenth century, Nicholas Culppeper, also herbolist and astrologer, declared it as "snake oil".

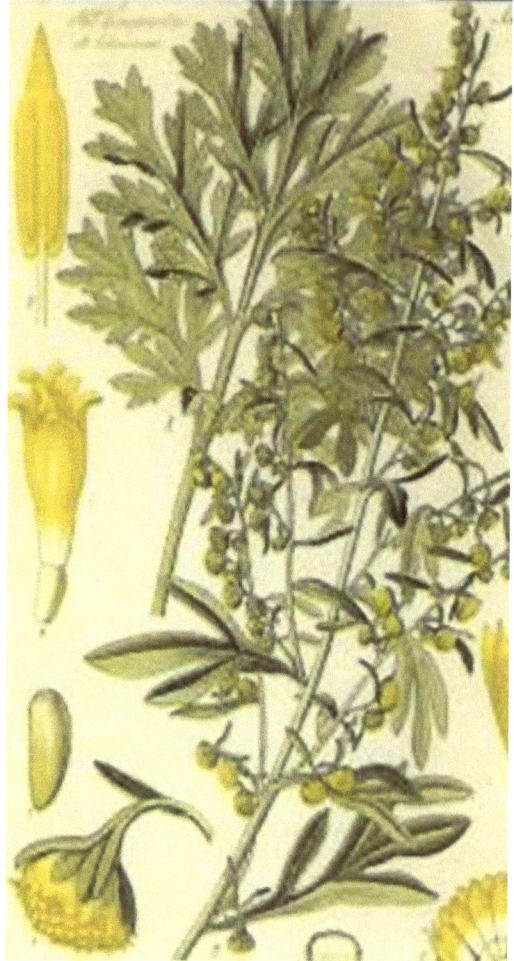

The modern Absinthe, a greenish distillate with a 65% of alcoholic content, appeared in the market in 1797 commercially produced by Henry Louis Pernod, who acquired the recipe of the Pierre Ordinaire, Swiss doctor of medicine recognized as a master in his profession. At a meteoric speed, thanks to a clever marketing, the consumption of Absinthe spread through western Europe, particularly in the Ville Lumière, ranking at the top of the social and political circles. Always present among the intelligentsia and the bohemia, The "Green Fairy" was becoming addicting, sometimes affecting important policy decisions with terrible results. It also affected the creative ability of literary giants such as Paul Verlaine, Charles - Guy de Maupassant, Victor Hugo, Oscar Wilde, Edgar Allan Poe and Ernest Dowson, among many others.

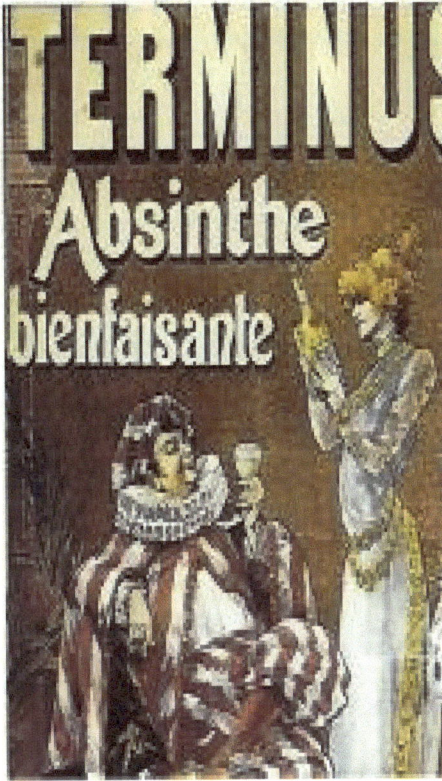

However no cultural field was more impacted by the "Fairy Green" than the impressionist painting style, fortunately in some cases, and fatally in others. Henry de Toulouse-Lautrec , Vincent Van Gogh, Edgar Degas, Edouard Manet, Paul Gauguin and Claude Monet became great friends at the time they took an "Abs" with a lump of sugar and cold water. The method for the consumption of Absinthe requires the use of a slotted spoon to maintain a lump of sugar over the drink and pouring cold water for its dissolution to counteract the bitter taste. This ritual was especially attractive, because until then all the alcoholic beverages were just ingested.

The manufacture of Absinthe was legally prohibited in Switzerland (1908), France (1915) and United States (1917). Reason: "Wormwood" is considered an addictive plant that can cause delirium, hallucinations and even mental impairment. Henry Pernod did not surrender, and after lengthy investigations, created a similar product: "La Petite Absente", the result of a substitution "Wormwood" by the "Southern Wormdwood", plant stripped of the botanical factors for which it was originally forbidden, producing a distillate of the same appearance.

Michael Roux of Crillon Importers, Inc., the pioneer importer of Vodka Absolut.

He presented to the world market Absinthe Refined, the version of our new era. With a content of 55% alcohol, it is delicious prepared with water and sugar, lemonade, seltzer water, lime juice and, if you have the temptation, prepare it in the original way, pouring a few drops of Absinthe over the lump of sugar and apply a slight flame. Film lovers can easily identify the "Fairy Green" in the movie **Moulin Rouge**.

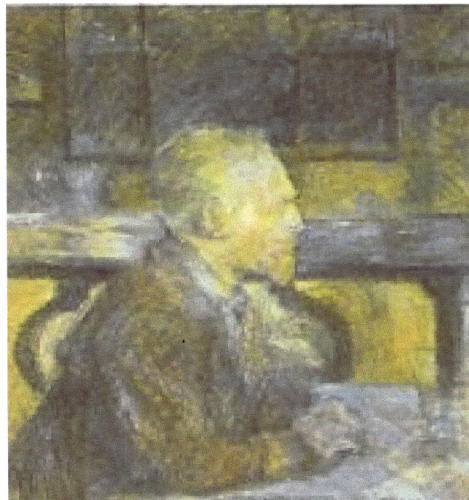

25

FROM BORDEAUX TO NAPA
Impressions on the two Wine "Mecas"

Bordeaux is not only the most famous region in the world of the art of grape growing, is also symbol of the Great Wines in general and a model for the universal enological industry. Pride of its natives can be perceived by the love of the grapevine culture exploring the beloved vineyards of their *terroirs*, culminated by the architectonic wonder of its Châteaux. The total production of its wines is equitably divided between red and white. The zone of the Médoc region, to the North, offers an extensive range of red wines considered "the glories of Bordeaux". The South part also provides to the consumer with good white wines, without reaching the excellence of the red ones, with the exception of the golden and sweet Sauternes, unique in its style.

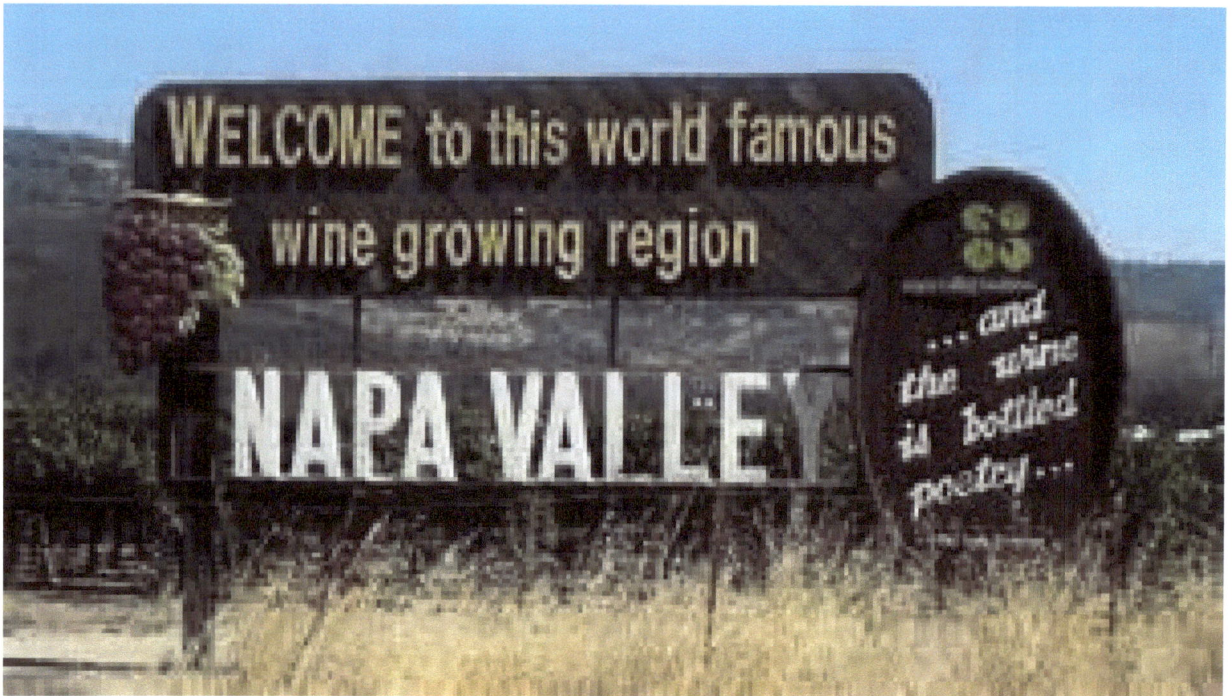

The Napa Valley is the standard of the Californian enological production and represents the commercial pinnacle of the industry in the United States. The diversity of climatic conditions creates different styles of wines. Nevertheless, all its grape growers share an agricultural characteristic in common, the power of absorption of the ground that prevents the saturation, something that can have disastrous consequences for the vineyards. The Pacific Ocean, to the East, covers an area celebrated, for its perennial subsoil deposits, influencing the ground to the point that one can identify presently more than 60 different types of *terroir*. The Chardonnays and Pinot Noirs, particularly those of the Carneros region are memorable. In certain areas of the Valley, mainly to the West, the volcanic subsoil of the "Great Ring of Fire" results in the production of a formidable red. Rough mountains and green hills of Napa allows the cultivation in terraces adorning the vineyard slopes.

In 1977, Peter Newton and his wife Su Hua settled in Spring Mountain acquiring 1 square mile of a hioll next to a fertile location in St. Helena, with a panoramic view of the Napa Valley. This is where the Newton Winery was born, producer of fine Bordeaux style reds and elegant typically Californian whites.

The grapevines, planted in high altitude terraces, between 500 and 1.600 feet above sea level, enjoy an ideal topography for their cultivation. The Newtons made use of all the ingredients necessary at their reach to conquer the top of the industry, obtaining the production of wines with the highest quality in the world.

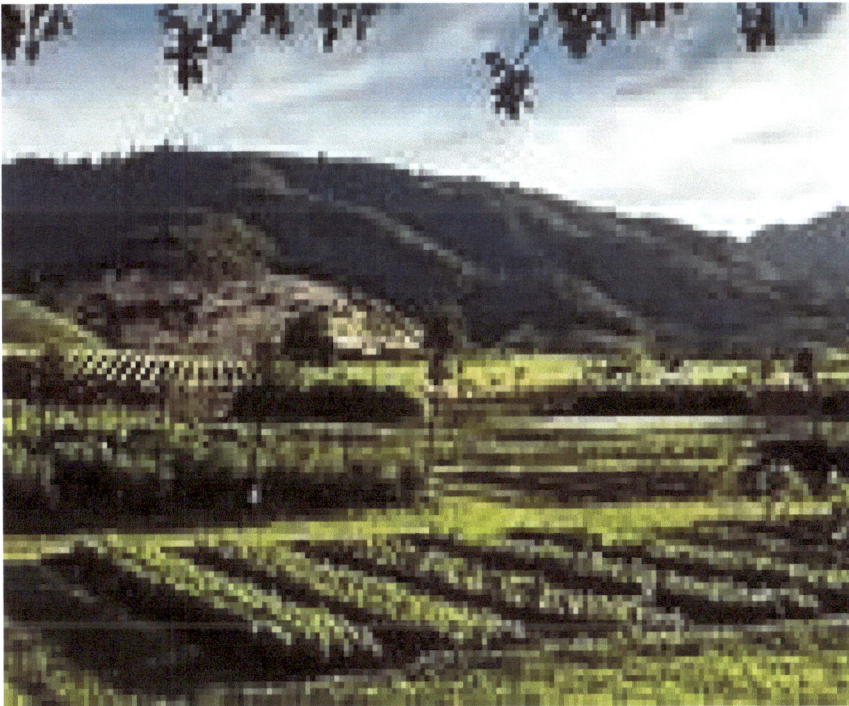

COLLECTION NEWTON WINERY:
Chardonnay 2004 (unfiltered)
Merlot 2002 (unfiltered)
Cabernet Sauvignon2002 (unfiltered)
Chardonnay 2004
Claret 2003– "The Puzzle"
The jewel of the collection (35%Cabernet Franc, 33% Cabernet Sauvignon, 23% Merlot, 9% Pétit Verdot).

THE MAGNIFICENT ENOLOGICAL LEGACY OF THE BENEDICTINE MONK DOM PERIGNON

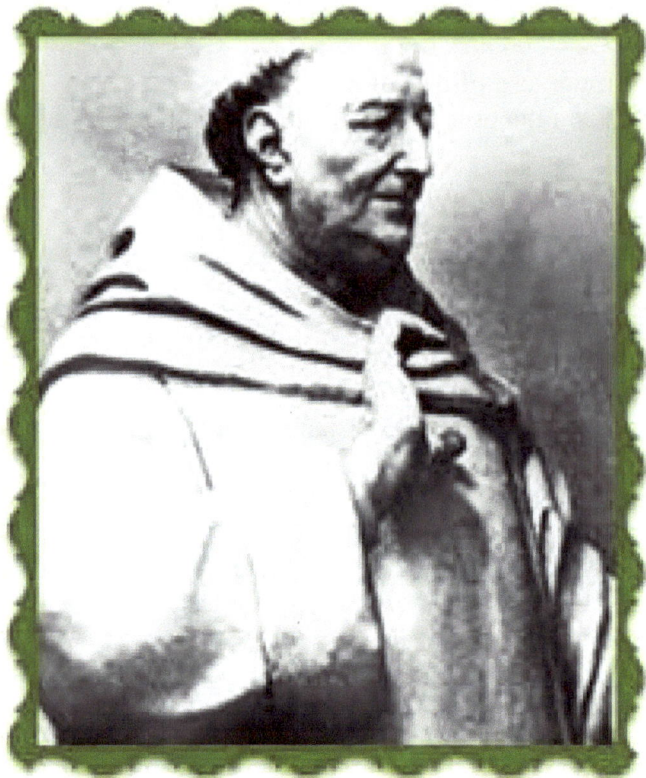

Returning almost fifteen centuries back, in the year 662, Archbishop Nivard, one of the Ecclesiastical authorities of more influence in France, ascended a hill in the heart of his native region of Champagne to appreciate "a vast and truly magnificent view" of the French countryside. Tired by the effort, he decided to rest seating in the shade of a shrub, and fell asleep for a while. In his dreams, Nivard saw a beautiful white dove flying in circles around the shrub where he rested. The Archbishop interpreted his dream to be a divine message asking him to build a sanctuary there, at the top of the hill. Thus the Abbey of Hautvillers emerged governed by the Order of Benedictine Monks for centuries, being the cradle of the most appreciated and elegant wine produced until the present time: The Champagne.

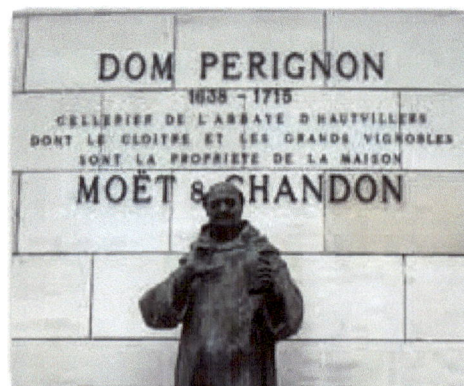

The 23rd of May 1668, the small Benedictine community of the Abbey gave welcome to a young monk called Pierre Pérignon, who in short time became responsible for the administration of the abbey, already well-known by its wines of great quality. Pierre, to whom his contemporaries knew by his religious surname Dom Pérignon, personally directed the warehouses of the Monastery, supervised the cultivation of the soil and often traveled by the region in charge of businesses, but he mostly enjoyed taking care and improving the vineyards. He was the first Master Winemaker of a cellar producing white wines coming from red grapes, obtaining a greater quality and character. The wines of the Abbey of Hautvillers of Pinot Noir and Chardonnay grapes, were legendary in all France for its perfect balance. A day in early summer, while he crossed the quiet Monastery warehouses, he observed a phenomenon. A certain number of bottles began to expel the cork spilling the wine noisly, surrounded by an effervescent sea. When asking one of his assistants, the person in charge of supervising the fermentation process, it was discovered that those wines, by accident, prematurely had been bottled without having completed their cycle in the barrel. Due to this accident a

28

powerful second fermentation ocurred in the bottle, incapable of retaining its content. Certain popular rosé sparkling wines already existed in the taverns of London, but nothing like the discovery that came out in Hautvillers. Dom Pérignon, confused, but intrigued by his curiosity, decided to taste such a wine. Hi was so impressed and delighted with the results that he stated "is a constellation of stars titillating in my palate". It was a huge finding of a wine to which Dom Pérignon would dedicate his enological experience.

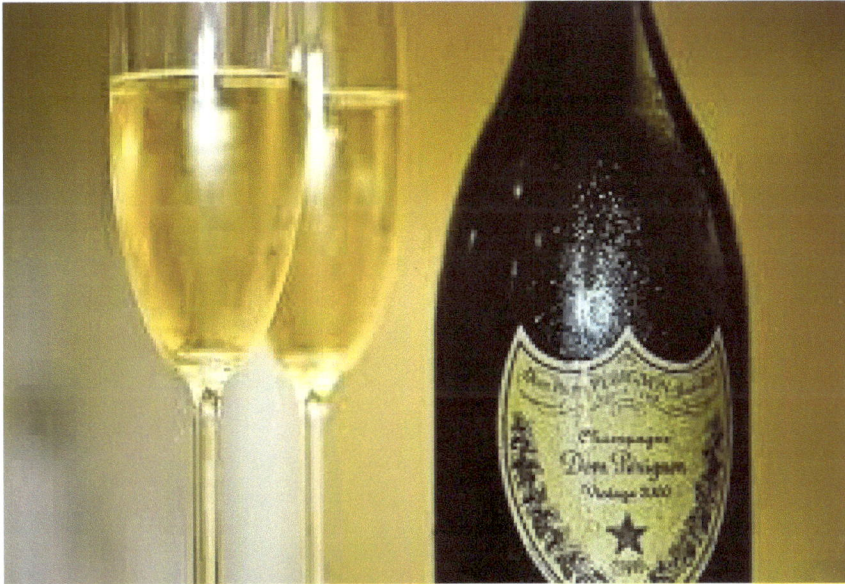

Louis XV, King of France received the first samples of the New Wine of Champagne from the Abbey of Hautvillers, making it know to the Court. It was a great event and even his concubine Madame Pompadour, expressed: "This erotic wine gives to women a powerful brilliance in the eyes and no redness in the cheeks like most others".

This unique sparkling wine made Pierre Dom Pérignon the spiritual father of Champagne and one of the great visionaries of the world of Wine.

On 1743 Claude Moet, wine merchant in Epernay, not very far from Hautvillers, founded his producing company of Champagne, presently characterized by his reputation for the respect of the past and nature. It was the initiative of his grandson, Jean-Remy Moet (1788-1841) to buy vineyards for new cultivations during the French Revolution. He established a new network of sales for export. During the years of the Empire, the company bloomed multiplying its production. By the end of the XIX century, the Moet & Chandon Champagne was well-known internationally.

As a great homage to the Pierre Dom Pérignon, the House of Moet & Chandon named this elegant *Tete de Cuvée* as **Dom Pérignon**, one of the best champagnes in the world.

ARRIVED FROM NEW ZEALAND

From the picturesque vineyards more South of the Globe

The historical chronicles on the appearance of New Zealand in the world map began with the discovery of the west coast of the North and South Islands in 1642 by the Dutch navigator Abel Jaszoon Tasman. His total circumnavigation tooh place between the years 1769 and 1770 under the leadership of James Cook, Admiral of the Royal British Navy. They were both in charge of the import of the first grapevines, of French origin.

It was not until the beginning of 1800s when the New Zealand table wines appeared for domestic consumption, initiating the intense cultivation of grapevines. Nevertheless the growth of the wine industry did not take place until the end of 1960s, concentrating in grape varieties coming from France, such as **Chardonnay, Sauvignon Blanc, Pinot Noir, Merlot and Cabernet Sauvignon.** The era of the modern vinificación, product promotion and opening of international markets began in 1985, setting the standard for the development of a wine industry of the fastest and most successful growth in contemporary History.

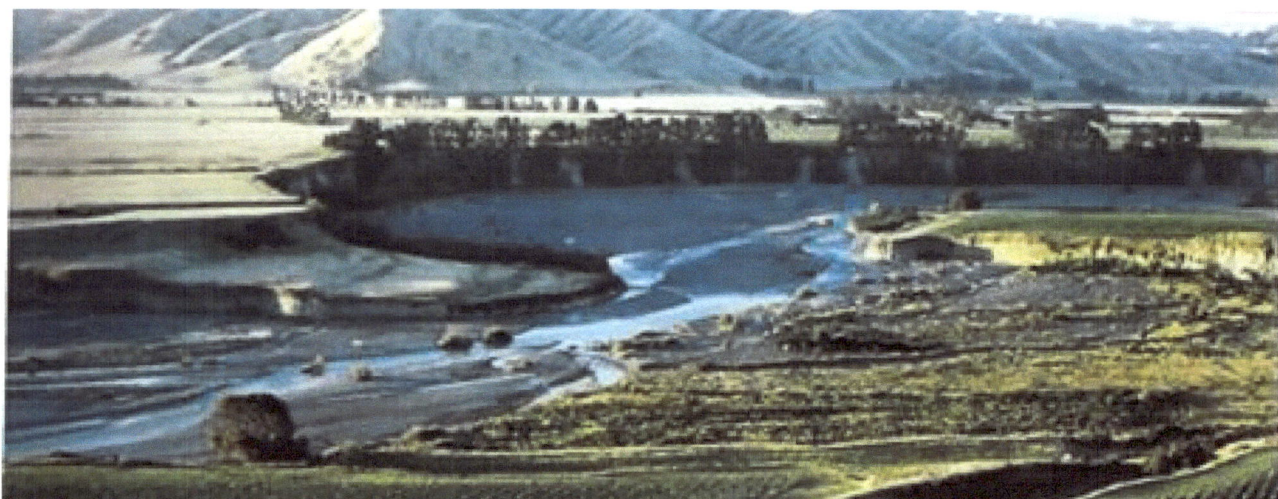

This great enological phenomenon marked the appearance of Sauvignon Blanc, coming originally from the Loire Valley. The New Zealand version fully exceeds the French style offering the consumer a refreshing white wine with the smooth aroma of citric fruits and great elegance. A festive and cheerful wine. Of similar form, the Chardonnay and the Pinot Noir, also of French ancestry, have their *"sui generis"* style, coming from the fresh and sunny climate of Marlborough, the region of greater industrial capacity and higher quality of production in the Islands. The New Zealand wine industry counts at the present time with more than 300 recognized producers, being **Stoneleigh** and **Brancot** wineries among the top of the industry with more than 30 years of history and world-wide recognition. Both wineries described the 2008 wine as an enological Prodigy.

These are their main characteristics:

STONELEIGH. Sauvignon Blanc 2008.
COLOR: Clear straw with emerald tones.
AROMA: Vibrant intensity of fruit. Mature pink grapefruit and passion fruit predominate.
BOUQUET: Mineral complexity in the palate, next to an excellent balance of mature fruit and fresh acidity. Great for sipping it alone or savoring with delicate white meats and seafood.

STONELEIGH. Pinot Noir 2007. COLOR: Light and crystalline ruby. AROMA: Black cherry, raspberry red plums and species. BOUQUET: A smooth and flexible wine with an end of sweet fruit and balanced tannins.

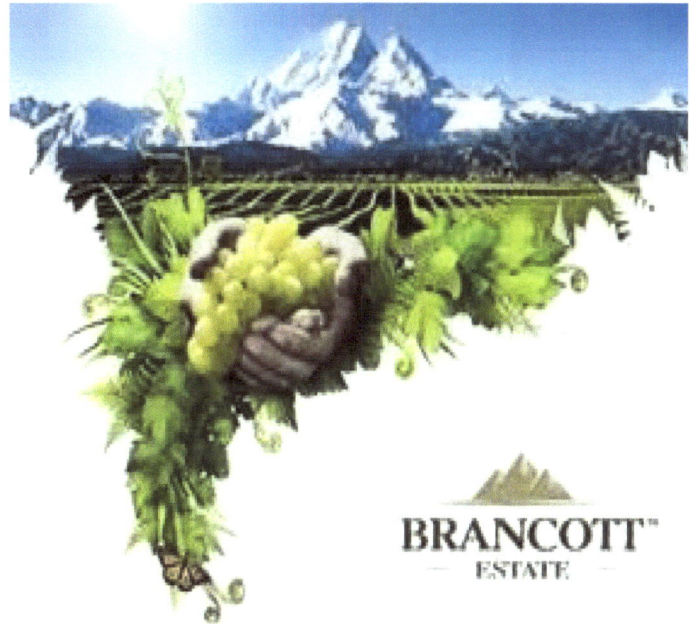

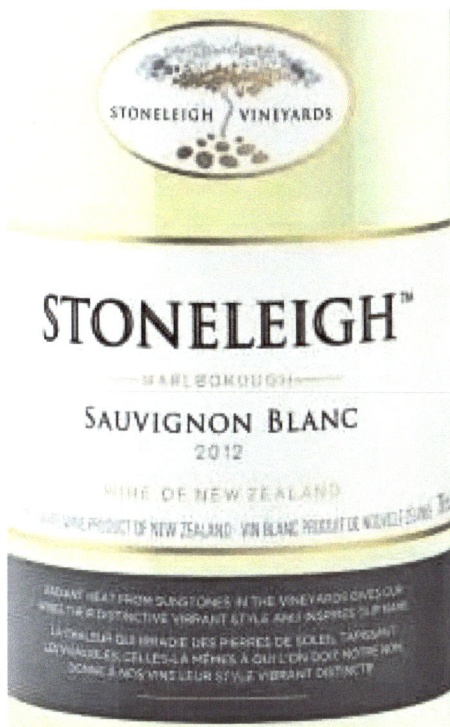

BRANCOTT Reserve Sauvignon Blanc 2008. COLOR: Pale straw with greenish tones. AROMA: Wild currant, *stone fruits* and red pepper. BOUQUET: Flavors of currant and fresh peach. Concentrated fruits balanced with tickling acidity. Delicious with all types of seafood.

BRANCOTT Reserve Pinot Noir 2007. COLOR: Crimson red. AROMA: Mature cherries and species accentuated by tones of fresh plum. BOUQUET: Denoting a red fruit and silky chocolate finale.

"The masterful owners of the wine cellasr of Brancott and Stoneleigh feel proud to share with the world the best of the 2008 wines of New Zealand", affirms Patrick Materman, head of the enologist team.

Welcome to Paradise!

THE RUM EMPIRE
Legendary, colorful, liturgical and festive a Spirit.

Rum, whose denomination originated in the English language as "rum", defines a spirit derived from the distillation of juice from sugar cane and molasses resulting from its fermentation. Obviously it is produced in all tropical geographic areas where sugar cane is cultivated.

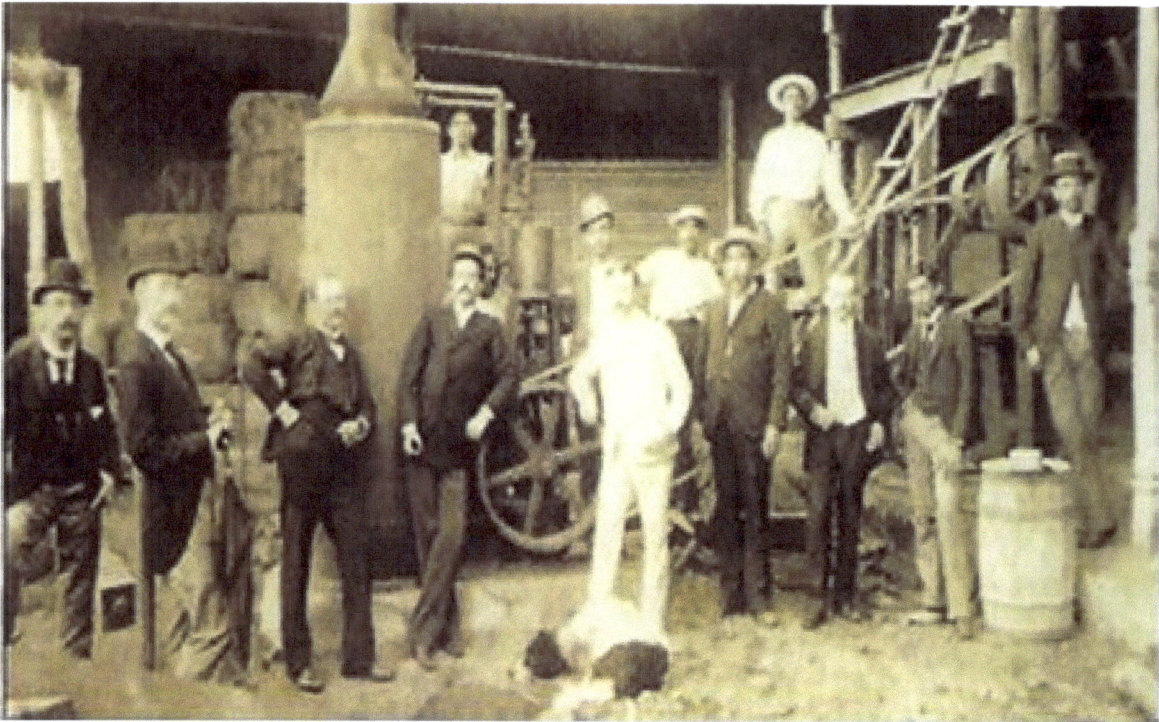

In the IV century B.C., Alexander the Great returned from his expedition to India, mentioning the powerful spirits extracted from sugar cane, which originated speculations of the existence of a "spirit" that fermented this juice naturally, without human intervention. The colonization vision of Cristopher Columbus was made once again apparent when in 1493, during his second expedition, made a stop in the Canary Islands bringing with him plantings of sugar cane, for its cultivation in Cuba and the Hispaniola..

In 1647, possibly before, Barbados bursted in with the distillation of rum baptized through the tropical countries as *"Waters of Barbados", "El Tumulto", "Muerte del Diablo", "Blood of Nelson"* (whose dead body was preserved in rum for his transfer to England) and with other nicknames unsuitable for publishing, coming from the hordes of pirates and buccaneers who infested the Caribbean. The British Empire visualized the potential impact in the international market, promoting an industrial production that internationalized the rum, overthrowing the gin in England like as the dominant distilled beverage. In 1655, the Royal English Navy included a half of pint of rum in the rations of its soldiers and combatants, while the distilleries proliferated in New York and

New England producing the spirit with molasses coming from of the Antilles. Exotic species of the Islands were integrated to perfume the product creating preferences and to perfume the liturgical rites of the religions of the African slaves.

In 1862, Don Facundo Bacardi Massó, Spanish immigrant from Catalonia, established a primitive distillery, the pillars of a future empire in Santiago de Cuba, where he developed a new formula for the production of a different rum, smoother and lighter than the fiery and spicy varieties of other Caribbean countries. The family name of distilling experts appeared in the labels of the product for the first time, opening the doors to more of a century of success in the Industry. Today the Bacardi name is considered internationally as a symbol of excellence enhancing the concept of the modern rum. Ideal for mixology or drink it straight. At the present time the Bacardi House produces an extensive range of rums, from the light White to the refined Reserve, also offering fruity based versions of lemon and orange.

Over a century ago, the main grower of sugar cane in Central America, the Pellas family, decided to distill rum to celebrate the *Zafra* or harvest as a joyful occassion. This celebration became a tradition commercialized in 1937 with the founding of the *Compañía Licorera* of Nicaragua. Its goal, to create a selection of rums of great quality, aged from 4 to 15 years, destined for export also creating a style of younger spirits for local consumption. The *Flor de Caña* rum was born! A great rum for sophisticated palates.

Recomendations:

GUATEMALA:
Ron Zacapa Centenario.
PUERTO RICO:
Ron del Barrilito – Captain Morgan.
JAMAICA: Myers/Appleton
DOMINICANA:
Barceló – Brugal. **BARBADOS:**
Mount Gay –
Malibu.
COLOMBIA:
Ron Viejo de Caldas. **VENEZUELA:**
Ron Pampero Aniversario.
AUSTRALIA:
Bundaberg.
USA: Great variety of creative tropical mixology based on rum. Louisiana and Alabama produce light rums of popular consumption.

THE NEW RON ATLANTICO
A Mixology tour from the heart of the Caribbean

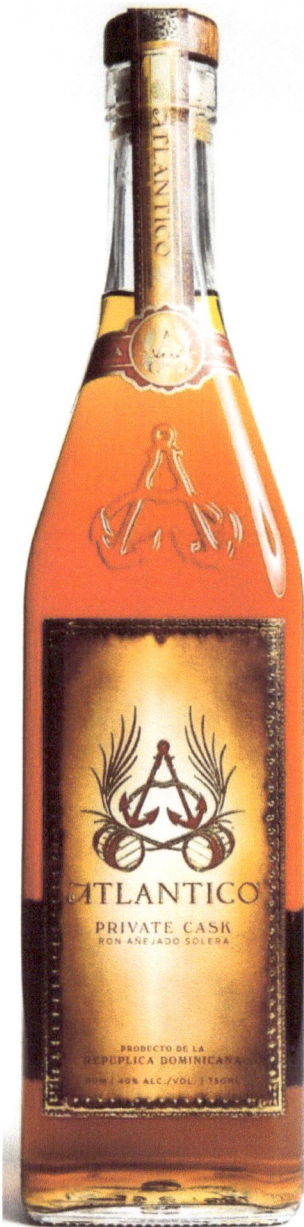

In 1493, during his second trip to the New World, Christopher Columbus brought with him from the Canary Islands the first plantings of sugar cane to promote its cultivation all along the Caribbean coasts.

Ron, Spanish for rum, according to most experts, originated in the Dominican Republic. There, amongst the lusciously forested mountains and large river valleys, sugar cane was first fermented into alcohol in the 17th century. Since then, the island is known for producing not only the best sugar cane in the world, but also the finest hand crafted rums, been the new ***Ron Atlántico Private Cask*** the greatest ambassador of them all.

Aleco Azqueta and Brandon Lieb, two spirits industry leaders who have managed some of the world's leading super premium brands, had a vision that turned into reality: the creation of the perfect rum reviving the classic cocktail culture. The process for ***Ron Atlántico*** begins with Aleco and Brandon handpicking the finest small batched aged rums in the island. Once selected, the rums are blended together under the watchful eye of the master blender, placed in small bourbon barrels (private cask) and aged again. This "marrying" system allows the different rums to interact with one another producing a more intriguing spirit. Then, the rum is removed from the "private casks" and placed into yet another set of barrels ageing once more, using the complex *solera* method, most typically used to produce sherry. In addition to scouting the best breeding grounds for their rum, Aleco and Brandon also wanted the best quality materials to package such creation.

Creative label design, the finest Italian glass bottles and refined cork closures from Portugal combined, offers to the consumer a "one of a kind" highly sophisticated finished product.

Ron Atlántico proudly presents to you a "do it yourself" recipe sample of classic Tropical Mixology.

Salud !

DAIQUIRI
2 oz. Ron Atlántico
1 oz. fresh lime juice
1 tsp. sugar
1 egg white

MOJITO
2 oz. Ron Atlántico
2 oz. club soda
12 mint leaves
1 tsp. sugar
1 oz. fresh lime juice

Shake vigorously all ingredients and strain in a cocktail glass.
Muddle mint leaves, sugar, lime juice, and float it on top.
Beat the egg white until creamy in a highball glass.
Add ice and Ron Atlántico stirring well.
Garnish with a slice of lime. Poor club soda and garnish with mint leaf.

HOT BUTTERED ATLANTICO (Serves 12)

1 stick unsalted butter
2 cups brown sugar
1 tsp. powered cinnamon
1 tsp. grated nutmeg
3 cloves
1 Btl. Ron Atlántico

Prepare a creamy mixture with the butter,
brown sugar, cinnamon, nutmeg, cloves & salt
in a medium size container. Refrigerate until
a firm consistence. Put 2 tablespoon of the reamy
mixture evenly divided into 12 tall glass cups.

Add 3 oz. of rum per serving and boiling water Boiling water & dash of salt to taste stirring well.
Garnish with cinnamon stick and serve immediately.

DOING JUSTICE TO THE SUBLIME WHITE WINE
An international reference to the best of the best

Many people ignore the excellence of the White Wine. The main reason is a massive inclination for the reds, due to its proprieties and health benefits, its great color, long ageing and that psychological sensation making people believe is more of "a drink" or a better pairing for a great cuisine. A mass of wine drinkers also believe white wines originate from white grapes and red wines come from red grapes. Nothing further from the truth. If

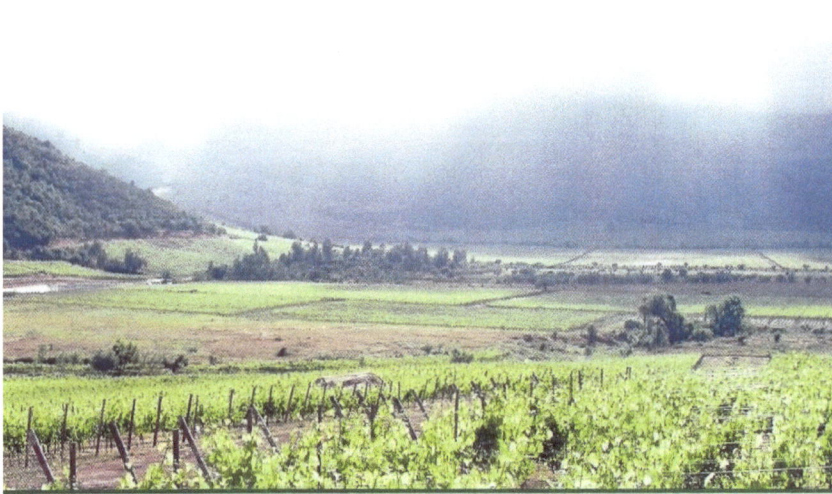
Outstanding view of the Chilean fields. Casa Lapostolle

we crush in our hand a white and a red grape together, we will realize the pulp's color is identical, only the skin keeps its red or light green tones. The skin in contact with the pulp marks the beginning of the *maceration process*, which brings up, according to the amount of time, the intensity in color. As a matter of fact, the golden *Champagne*, King of the wines, is a blend of the white grape Chardonnay with the Pinot Noir and Pinot Meunier varieties, both red. We want to enjoy the youth and freshness of white wines. Cooler climates are best for their *terroir*. Apples, pears, peaches and citric fruits are the foundation of its aromas and bouquets. Is advisable not to keep them for more than 9 or 10 years, unless you run into an outstanding vintage, which can last 20 years in good shape. However, we recommend to open most whites within the first 4 or 5 years. The turning of color will tell you. Enjoy them chilled, but do not go over 45 degrees, you will erase some of its bouquet. We are going to elaborate on examples of the most significant white wines of Europe, U.S.A., Oceania and South America, mainly emphasizing the most noble of the varieties *The Chardonnay.*

GERMANY: The Federal Republic is the largest producer of white wines in the world. Riesling, Muller-Thurgau and Silvaner grapes cover more than 50% of its land, offering wines mostly demi-sec and sweet. The wine laws in Germany are based on sugar and alcohol contain called *distinctions*. We recommend the following: *Kabinet* (demi-sec), *Spatlese* (late harvest), *Auslese*, (select harvest) and *Doktor* (smoothly dry). Great with any white fish and, believe it or not, fantastic for barbecues.

FRANCE: We all know *Champagne* is the Royal sparkling white wine of France. Its birth was nothing but a cellar accident due to an excess of yeast in a bottle fermentation process discovered by the monk Dom Pérignon, cellar master of the Abbey of Hautevillers in the Champagne region. As table wine our recommendations are the Chardonnays from the Burgundy region *(Le Montrachet))* and the Sauvignon Blancs from the Loire Valley (*Chateau Sancerre*).

ITALY: *Pinot Grigio, Soave, Orvieto, Verdicchio* and *Asti* are the most popular white wines in Italy. Full of a smooth dryness make excellent table wines. However, let's not forget Italy is, regarding production and consumption, a red wine country.

SPAIN: The Rias Baixas region, in the northwest of the country, produces the *Albariño* wine, one of the best in Europe (*Martin Códax*). Of course, we can't omit to mention the spirited *Vino de Jerez*, "the Sun of Spain in a bottle". Sherry and Manzanilla are part of the Spaniard's heart. *Casa Osborne* and *Lustau* are the best in the market.

U.S.A. : The champion white grape in the United States is without a doubt the *Chardonnay* variety. Particularly the California Chardonnay wines differ from the rest of the world in style. You can find the straw pale dry in the areas close to the Pacific coast, Sonoma, Monterrey, and Santa Barbara (*Sonoma Coutrer, Gloria Ferrer)* and the fruit intense, golden color Chardonnays in Napa Valley, near the desert (*Newton, Domain Chandon).*

OCEANIA: What Australia and New Zealand have achieved in little more than 20 years of their wine history is miraculous. A monumental winemaker's emigration in the 60s opened the doors to the production of some of the greatest wines in the market, holding a spectacular value.

The greatest Chardonnay wines come from Australia, sourced from the best vineyards of the Victoria region (*Green Point)*, while the most joyful and festive Sauvignon Blanc (*Cloudy Bay)*are produced in New Zealand.

SOUTH AMERICA: Due to the Spanish conquest, the ***Vitis Vinifera*** grape was present in most Latin American regions in the XVI century, thriving in Argentina and Chile above all countries.

Their geographical position, south of the Tropic of Capricorn, insures an almost perfect climate well suited to viticulture. In particular, the slopes of the Andes provide the ideal terrain, complemented by ample sunshine, dry heat, cooling breezes and irrigations waters from melted snow feeding a great number of rivers. As a result, South America today is the second most important wine-producing continent after Europe. The Chardonnay wines, of a Californian style, we'll like to recommend are *Terrazas de los Andes* (Argentina) and *Casa Lapostolle* (Chile).

It's not only red what glitters !

WINE WONDERS OF NEW ZEALAND

The Marlborough region and Brancott Estate presents "Flight Song"

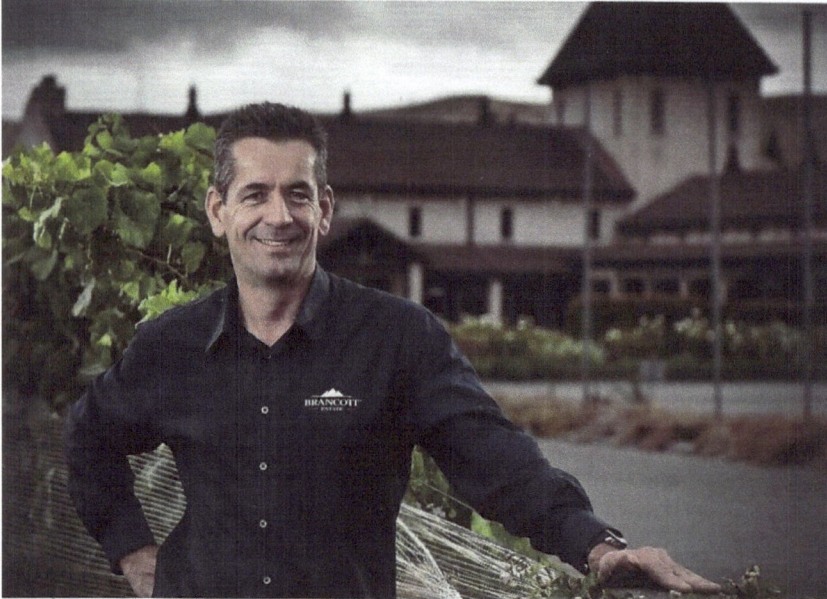

Patrick Materman. Chief Winemaker

Wine making and vine growing go back to colonial times in New Zealand. British Resident and keen oenologist James Busby was, as early as 1836, attempting to produce wine at his land in Waitangi. In 1851 French Roman Catholic missionaries in Hawke's Bay established New Zealand's oldest existing vineyard. Due to economic and cultural factors, such as animal agriculture, legislation favoring temperance and an overwhelming predominance of beer and spirit drinking, wine was for many years

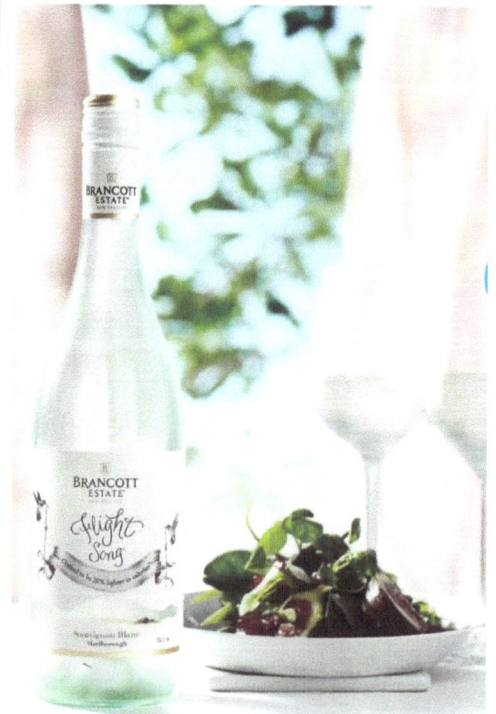

a marginal activity in terms of economic importance. Dalmatians immigrants arriving in New Zealand at the end of the nineteenth and beginning of the twentieth century, brought with them viticultural knowledge and planted vineyards in West and North Auckland. Typically, their vineyards produced sherry and port for the palates of the New Zealanders of the time, and table wine for their own community. However, great changes were forthcoming. In 1973, Britain entered the European Economic Community, which required the ending of historic trade for New Zealand opening the door to the viticultural activity. The late 1960s and early 1970s noted the rise of the "overseas experience", where young New Zealanders traveled, lived and work overseas predominantly in Europe. As a cultural phenomenon, the "overseas" experience predates the rise of New Zealand's premium wine industry under the European influence.

In the 1970s, the region of Marlborough started producing wines which were labeled by year of production (vintage) and grape variety following the style of wine producers in Australia. The first production of a Sauvignon Blanc, New Zealand's most illustrious wine, appears to have occurred in 1977. Also produced in that year were superior quality wines such as

Riesling, Cabernet Sauvignon and Pinotage rise highly the consumption with a great local interest and pride. Marlborough is one of the regions of New Zealand, located in the northeast of the South Island, named after the famous soldier and stateman, the Duke of Marlborough. The region is known for its dry climate, the picturesque Marlborough Sounds and Sauvignon Blanc wines and can claim the starting of the modern New Zealand wine industry.

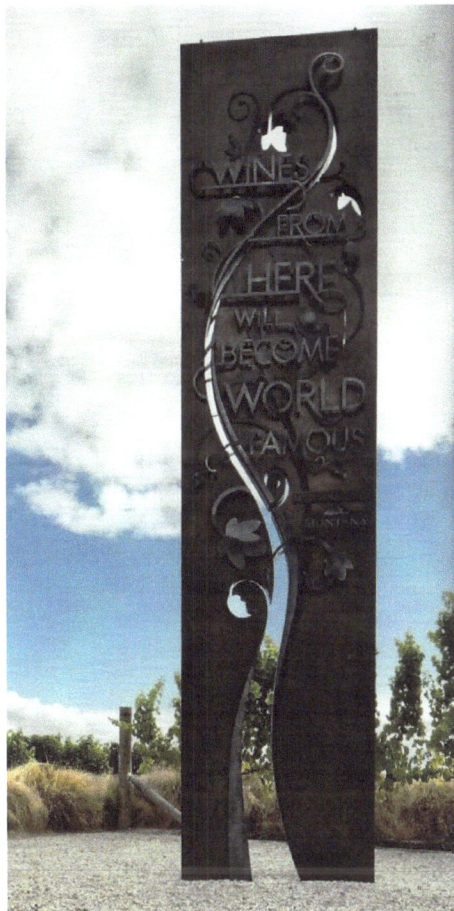

Wine lovers now have the freedom to enjoy the full flavor of the original Marlborough Sauvignon Blanc with Brancott Estate "Flight Song". As their Pinot Grigio the wines have been crafted to be 20% lighter in calories retaining its freshness and ripe flavors.
Presenting:

FLIGHT SONG. Sauvignon Blanc 2013: From early harvested grapes. The fruit was gently pressed before being fermented in a number of stainless steel tanks with a variety of yeasts types. Ferments were at cool temperatures to retain the very distinctive regional and varietal characters. The wine shows fragrant lemongrass aromas with almost pungent tomato leaf intensity. On the palate, the sweetness of these flavors is balanced with grapefruit-like acidity. Made to drink upon release while still young and exuberant, but could be cellared for up to two years from release. Best served chilled, you can enjoy this Sauvignon Blanc on its own or with a variety of foods from delicate to spicy grilled or barbecued seafood to green salads and Mediterranean dishes. Alcohol content: 9.0%

FLIGHT SONG Pinot Grigio 2013: The grapes were harvested from mid to late March 2013.
Brancott Estate followed with this wine the very same process of fermentation than its Sauvignon Blanc. Serve chilled and keep it for two years in the cellar if desired. On the nose, the wine shows an array of sweet fruit aromatics from guava to melon supplemented with ripe golden kiwifruit and nashi pear notes. These fresh fruit flavors combine on the palate to create a fullness with ripe golden delicious apple-like acidity to create balance. Enjoy this Pinot Grigio on its own, with delicate or spicy white meats and seafood dishes through to salads and cheeses. Alcohol content: 9.0%

"The fruit flavor and balance of these wines continually astounds me"
Patrik Materman. Chief Winemaker

O VINHO DO PORTO, GLORY OF PORTUGAL
A microcosm of the Wine World.

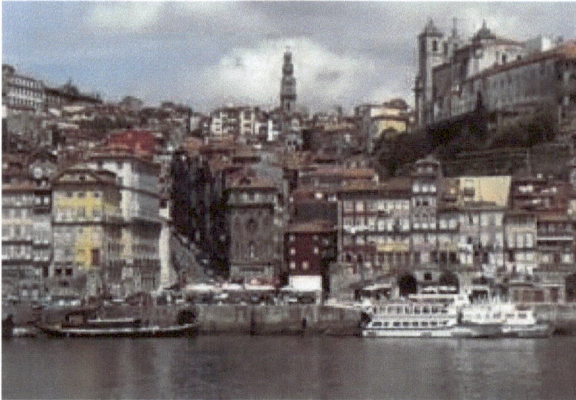

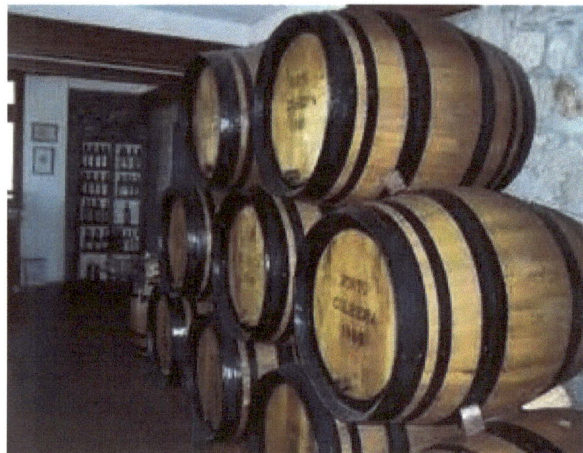

Portugal is the most appropriate place for a romantic wine enjoyment . Yet beyond Italy. Is the country of the ox-thrown squeaking carts carrying the plump clusters, the sunlight filtering through the grapevines, the moving about of the magic purple juice, the young girls carrying jars full of fortified nectars and the melancholic songs passed on throughout the centuries.

Today, the direct descendants of Portugal's seafarers and explorers are beginning to discover the high value of their wine estates (QUINTAS) in the Douro river valley, the most imposing, intensive and wildest wine-growing landscape anywhere. Its geological terrace-like vineyards call for the most primitive methods of hand collection and transportation on donkeys, mules and on someone's back until reaching a track suitable for wheeled transport. With an amazing dynamism and fueled by the European Union exporting development

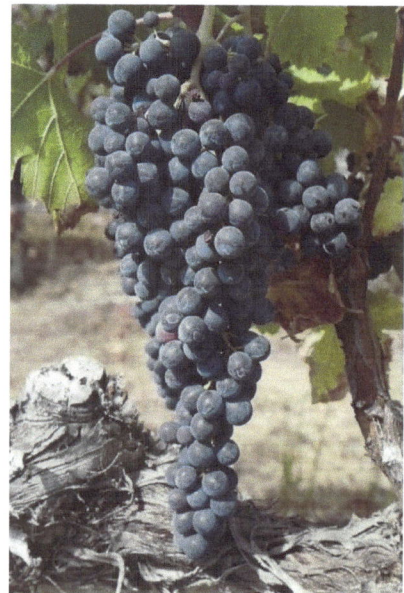

programs, the historically minded Portuguese are exploiting the potential of their vineyards, and the country long winemaking traditions to the full. Portugal is often described as the holder of the greatest variety of grapes in the world – supposedly 500 of them –, which is indeed amazing. Many can be assumed to have their origins far back in the Middle Ages – the XII century – in the golden times of the monasteries and their viticulture.

Without a doubt, Portugal's finest wine – the one with the greatest character and unique style in existence – is the sophisticated Oporto, the only wine in the world served from right to left.

It is also simply known as Port or Vinho do Porto, beign named not after its place of origin but after

Porto, the harbor from which it is shipped all over the world. Its twin town Vila Nova de Gaia, on the opposite side of the Douro River is where the majority of port wines still lie today, maturing and aging for very long periods in the cellars of the coldest slopes of the region. There exist three basic types of Porto wines; White Porto: made with white grapes. We find them dry, medium dry or sweet; Ruby Porto: Intense, powerful, full-bodied wines. Tawny Porto: More evolved wines, lighter, charged with red fruits and spiced aromas; the best for aging. Port alcohol content is of about a 20% and its silky sweet bouquet is a caress in the palate. Full of dry fruit, berry and nut flavors we definitely recommend all three styles to enjoy them with friends, with family or when relaxing alone. They are succulent chilled as an aperitif, accompanying luscious desserts – especially if chocolate is involved – or simply "solo". Something very important to have in mind: Oporto should always be decanted.

We want to elaborate on three extraordinary brands, accessible in the USA and Latin American markets:
 RAMOS PINTO: Founded in 1880 by Adriano Ramos Pinto is a unique port coming from a property of extensive vineyards in the most favored sites of the Douro region. This allows it to have total control of grape production of their many brands. Among them Porto Fine White – Porto Vintage 2003 – Quinta do Bom Retiro, 20 years Tawny and The Collector, Ruby Reserva.

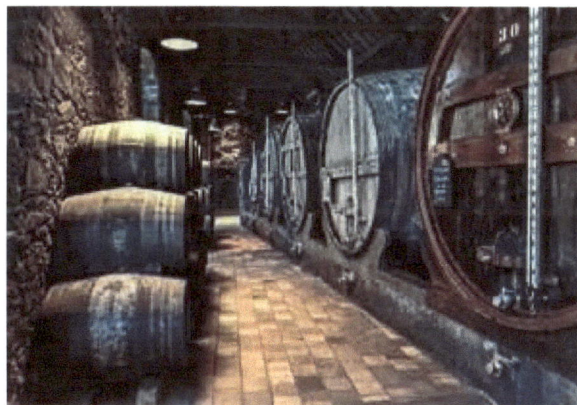

SANDEMAN: With a loan of 300 sterling pounds, George Sandeman – a young ambitious Scotsman – rented a cellar in 1790 and initiated a wine business in the City of London. Later on founded his own enterprise – George Sandeman & Co. – and by 1810 he started operations in Portugal and Spain which have developed in to today's impressive Porto lodges and Sherry bodegas. Always with the world-export idea in mind.

The jewels of the collection: Vau Vintage 2000 – Founders Reserve – Tawny Porto, 20 Years Old and Tawny Porto, 40 Years Old.

 COCKBURN'S: The company was founded in 1815 and has grown to become one of the world's great port houses. Makers of a complete line of fine ports, Cockburn's is known worldwide for its mature, slightly drier wine style signature and also is the largest vineyard owner in the Port district. Their wood aged ports are blended wines from multiple vintages which means they should be enjoyed upon release. Choose one of the following or, better yet, try them all: Special Reserve – Cockburn's Fine Ruby – Cockburn's Fine Tawny – LBV, Late Bottled Vintage – 10 Year Old Tawny – 20 Year Old Tawny – Quinta dos Canais – Vintage Port.

A romantic trip to Oporto, tasting its wines, will do wonders for you !

AN ITALIAN MARVEL

Capezzana. Tuscany's most revered wines.

Not only is Italy the top wine producing country in the world, it is also one of Europe's oldest producers.

Recent archeological finds have shown that the vine was systematically cultivated in Italy by the Etruscans in the 8th century B.C. We can assume that efforts were maid to cultivate the vine even earlier, though clear proof of this has not yet been established. The Etruscans brought viticulture and wine industry to perfection, and their achievements became a model. With the advent of the Roman Empire advanced skills and expertise in vine cultivation and winemaking spread throughout Western and Central Europe. The Romans were also responsible for the development of wine trade into a very profitable economic activity, due to, among other customs, the religious cult to Bacchus, the Roman variant of the Greek God Dionysus. With the rise of Christianity and up to its recognition as a state religion in the 4th century, the consumption of wine, in the context of cult activities became more moderate. However, the time passed and winemaking was a part of life itself. Some of the brand names which are still well known in the world of wine today were established as early as the 13th and 14th centuries in Central Italy, been Tuscany and its Florentine nobility associated to the art of viticulture. Records dated in 804 reveal that vines were cultivated at the Capezzana estate. 1200 years later this region is producing some of the greatest supertoscans for today's wine lovers.

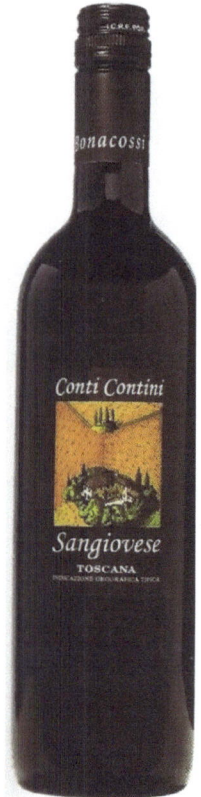

In the 1920's Count Alessandro Contini Bonacossi bought the Capezzana estate, divided into three parts and incorporating more than 120 farms producing high quality wines and olive oil, been later further improved and enlarged through significant work and investment. Capezzana is situated in northern Tuscany, in the commune of Carmignano, just 20 Km. from Florence. Today, this noble wine estate is in an almost unique position of having bottles of vintages dating from 1925. The property has 670 hectares comprising a Medici villa, and an adjacent farm with historic cellars beneath it, dating from the 16th century. Summer daytime temperatures are high and nights are cool on account of the winds off the Apennines mountains.

Recorking old vintages, a delicate and complex process

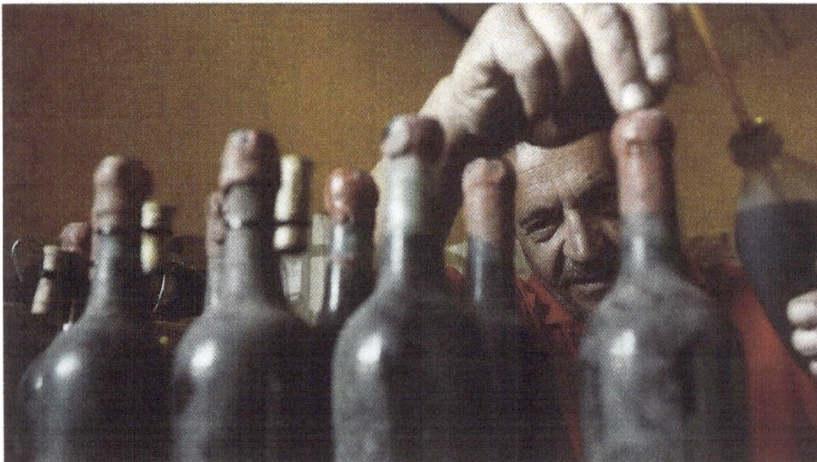

These conditions ensure good maturing of the grapes, which are generally one to two weeks ahead of all the other Tuscan wine-growing regions. Let's elaborate about these unique wines:

42

TREBBIANO DI CAPEZZANA 2001 (100% Trebbiano): COLOR: Yellow-amber with green nuances. NOSE: Aromas of almond, yellow flowers and vanilla – PALATE: Intense, harmonic, well balanced with a long and persistent finish – RECCOMENDATIONS: White meats and cheese.

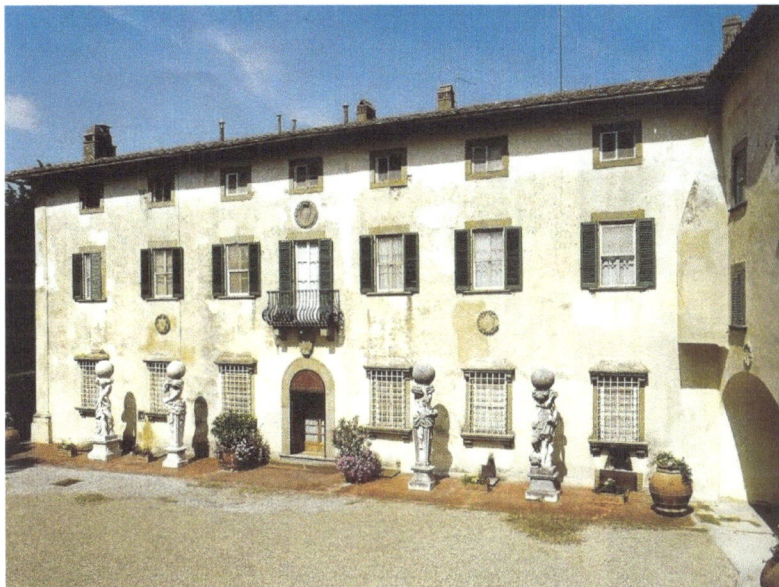

CHARDONNAY TOSCANA 2008 (100% Chardonnay): COLOR: Canary yellow with light reflections tending to green – NOSE: Fruity, with tones of sweet fruits, white, and yellow flowers – PALATE: Full-bodied, soft with fruit, lasting finish.
RECOMMENDATIONS:
Excellent aperitif, good with first courses in general and fish main courses.

TREFIANO 1999 (80 Sangiovese – 10% Cabernet Sauvignon – 10% Canaiolo): COLOR: Ruby red, Intensely purplish. NOSE: Ample, elegante, persistent, fruity with sweet and spicy Suances – PALATE: Soft, rich in texture, opulent with firm tannins. Well balance acidity, harmonious texture and body. Long, Persistent finish with a combination of red berries and spices. RECOMMENDATIONS: Game, white and red meats and cheese.

Campezzana also produces extra virgin olive oil, made mainly from Moraiolo and Frantoio olives with a small percentage of Pendolino and Leccino varieties

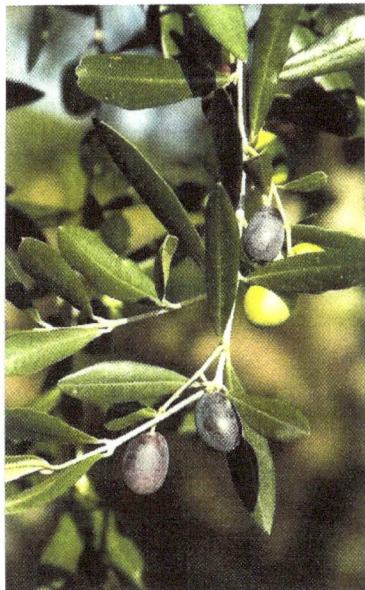

BARCO REALE (70% Sangiovese – 20% Cabernet Sauvignon – 10% Canaiolo): COLOR: Deep red with a purple touch and ruby red shades – NOSE: Sweet, round, elegant, very intense fruit with light tones of oak. – PALATE: Soft, voluminous, ample with sweet tannins of medium density in good balance with the acidity. Fruity, sweet, long lasting finish. RECOMMENDATIONS: Most pasta dishes. White and red meats.

CONTE CONTINI TOSCANA 2007 (100% Sangiovese): COLOR: Ruby red, garnet red shades – NOSE: Ample, fine, ethereal, fruity with sweet and spicy nuances. PALATE: Soft, good texture and sweet tannins. Well balanced with a red fruit and spicy finish. RECOMMENDATIONS: Most meats and cheeses.

VILLA DI CAPEZANNA 2001 (80% Sangiovese – 20% Cabernet Sauvignon): COLOR: Deep ruby red. NOSE: Ample, elegant, refined, sweet and fruity with spicy aromas. PALATE: Soft, firm with dense and Sweet tannins. Well balanced acidity with harmonious texture and body.

43

Long an persistent finish with spicy tones. RECOMMENDATIONS: Red and white meats and most types of cheeses.

GHIAIE DELLA FURBA 2000 (70% Cabernet Sauvignon – 20% Merlot – 10% Syrah): COLOR: Intense and impenetrable ruby red. NOSE: Ample, complex, elegant, sweet, fruity, intensely spicy. PALATE: Sweet, firm and full-bodied. Quite opulent with dense, sweet tannins. Well balance and a long finish with persistent fruitiness of wild berries and spicy tones. RECOMMENDATIONS: Red meats, game, hard seasoned cheese.

VIN RUSPO – ROSATO DI CARMIGNANO (80 Sangiovese – 10% Cabernet Sauvignon – 10 Canaiolo) COLOR: Lively rosé. NOSE: Fruity, sweet, ample and clean. PALATE: Soft, light body, harmonic and well balanced acidity. Fruity finish. RECOMMENDATIONS: An excellent entry wine. Great with first courses and white meats.

VINSANTO DI CARMIGNANO RISERVA 2003 (90% Trebbiano – 10% San Colombano): COLOR: Deep golden yellow. NOSE: Complex with dried fruit, candied apricot and orange peel aromas. Yellow Flowers nuances. PALATE: Sweet, soft and opulent with a sweet, persistent finish of candied fruit.
RECOMMENDATIONS: All desserts.

We also want to suggest trying CAPEZZANA OLIO DI OLIVA EXTRAVIRGINE. Extraordinary!

Enjoy history, tradition and family care in each sip!

Capezzana combines tradition with modern techniques to create truly remarkable wines

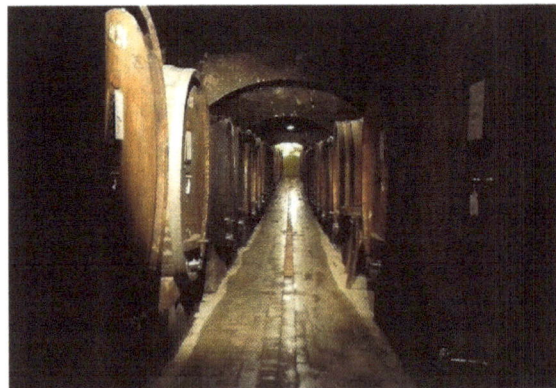

The Capezzana Estate historical cellars date back to the Sixteenth century, and are still preserved today as a testimony of the rich history of the property

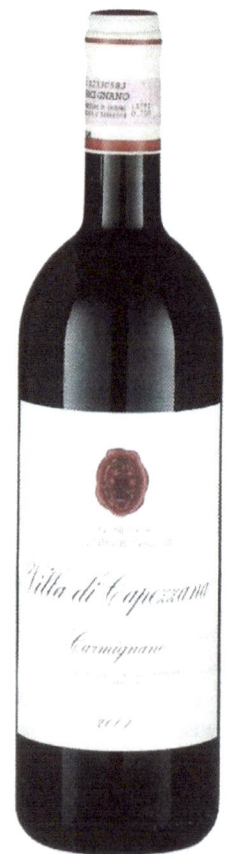

A LEGENDARY WINE DINASTY FROM JEREZ

González Byass, a family internationally renowned in the Industry

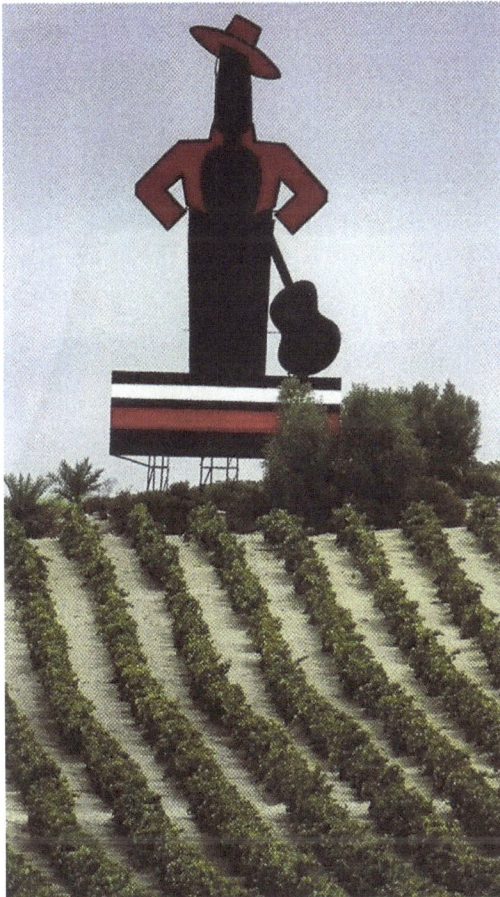

Don Manuel Maria González Angel (1812-1887), at the young age of 23, decided that he wished to be part of the prosperous and thriving business of wines. Advised by his uncle, José Angel de la Peña – who became the famous Tío Pepe ("Uncle Joe" acclaimed as the finest Sherry in existence) – Don Manuel founded the company that is today one of the largest and most diversified wine business in the world, particularly symbolizing the spirit of the Land of Jerez for more than 175 years, beginning with the first order sent to London from his bodegas: 10 barrels of Vino de Jerez, 62 barrels the following year and 406 barrels by 1839. It was then when the company began its relationship with Robert Blake Byass, from the London firm Byass & Carrington, merchants of great reputation and buyers of sherry from other companies in Jerez. With this new partnership, the sales grew year after year, entering in new markets such as France, Germany and even as far as Russia.

The world famous brand, Tío Pepe, dates from 1844 and is not only the most sold Fino sherry throughout the world but also the Spanish product present in the highest number of countries in the world.

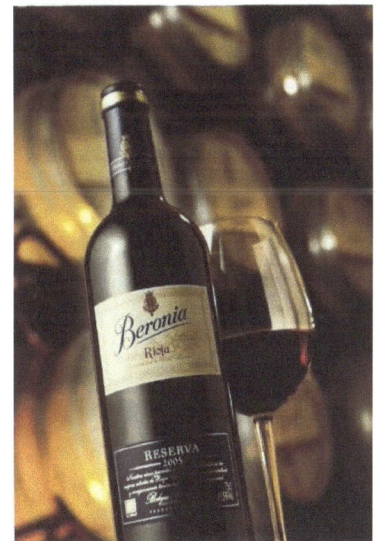

From then on Don Manuel's vision led him to extend his wine & spirits business, becoming in 1863 the company "González Byass" exporting sherry wines from Jerez at a volume of 3,885 barrels, the equivalent to 2,590.000 bottles. At the same time Don Manuel had set modern stills in order to obtain wine liquor to be used in the production of brandy, applying the traditional technique of "solera" y "criadera" used in the ageing process, utilizing the same barrels which had previously contained wine. In 1963 the Gran Bodega Tío Pepe was constructed, with three floors, a roof consisting of four concrete domes, and a capacity for 30,000 barrels. After a "non stop" rapid development, in 1985, the 150 anniversary of the company, González Byass received the highest distinction from the Town Council of Jerez, "La Medalla de Oro de la Ciudad" ("The Gold Medal of the City") for its contribution to the development of Jerez. The business continues to be managed by the Gozález family with direct descendants of Don Manuel Maria (fifth generation)

45

holding management positions.   González Byass, the most ambitious wine & spirits enterprise today, has in the world market a portfolio of 79 different products coming from the most celebrated Spain's wine regions.

Let us elaborate:

Vinos de Jerez: Tío Pepe: Fino. 100% Palomino variety – Viña AB: Amontillado. 100% Palomino – Leonor: Palo Cortado. 100% Palomino – Alfonso: Dry oloroso. 100% Palomino – Cristina: Sweet oloroso. 87% Palomino, 13% Pedro Ximenez – Solera 1847: Sweet Oloroso. 75% Palomino, 25% Pedro Ximenez – Néctar PX:100% Pedro Ximenez - : Croft: Pale Cream. 100% Palomino – Del Duque: Amontillado. 100% Palomino – Apóstoles: Palo Cortado. 100% Palomino – Matusalem: Sweet oloroso. 75% Palomino, 25% Pedro Ximenez – Noé: 100% Pedro Ximenez – Añada 1982: Palo Cortado. 100% Palomino.

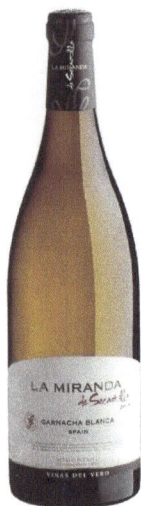

Vinos de Rioja: Beronia: One of the most distinguishes brands of this region. La Rioja is considered the top producer of Spain in quantity and quality alike. Gonzalez Byass presents 12 different Beronia brands:

Viura , white – Barrel Fermented Viura – White – Rosado, Rosé. 95% of Beronia are red winess: Crianza. 100% Tempranillo grape – Reserva and Gran Reserva. Tempranillo, Graciano y Mazuelo varieties – Beronia Graciano. 100% Graciano grape. – Reserva Mazuelo. 100% Mazuelo grape – Tempranillo

Special Production. 100% Tempranillo grape – Beronia Ecológico. Organic. 100 Tempranillo grapes – 198 Barricas. Tempranillo, Graciano and Mazuelo grapes. - Beronia III a.C. Tempranillo, Graciano and Mazuelo grapes. Limited production Assorted Wine Regions: Tierra de Castilla: Finca Constancia y Altozano (Toledo) – Cava y Penedés. Villa Arnau (Barcelona) – Tierra de Cádiz: Finca Moncloa (Andalucía) – Somontano: Viñas del Viero (Aragón).

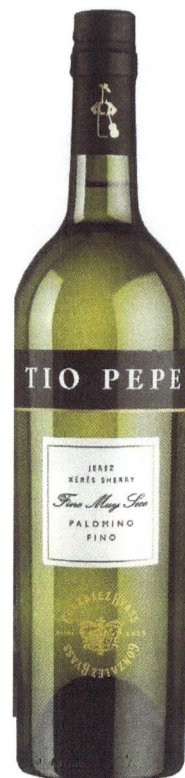

Liquors and Spirits: Brandies de Jerez: *Solera.* **Soberano – Solera** *Gran Reserva.* **Lepanto – Anís Chinchón** Sweet/Dry – **Gin**. **London No. 1 – Verotza** : Caramel Liqueur – **Granpecher:** Peach Liqueur
Granpomier: Apple Liqueur.

Oils and Vinegars: Bottled under the property name label: *Hacienda de Bracamonte.* Extra Virgin Olive Oil. Jerez Vinegar. Jerez Vinegar Reserva. Pedro Ximenez Vinegar.

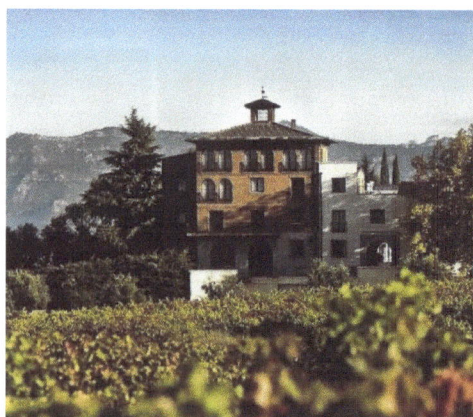

Let's toast on five generations of wisdom ¡

THE CALIFORNIA GIANT

The legacy of the great *Robert Mondavi* to the American wine industry

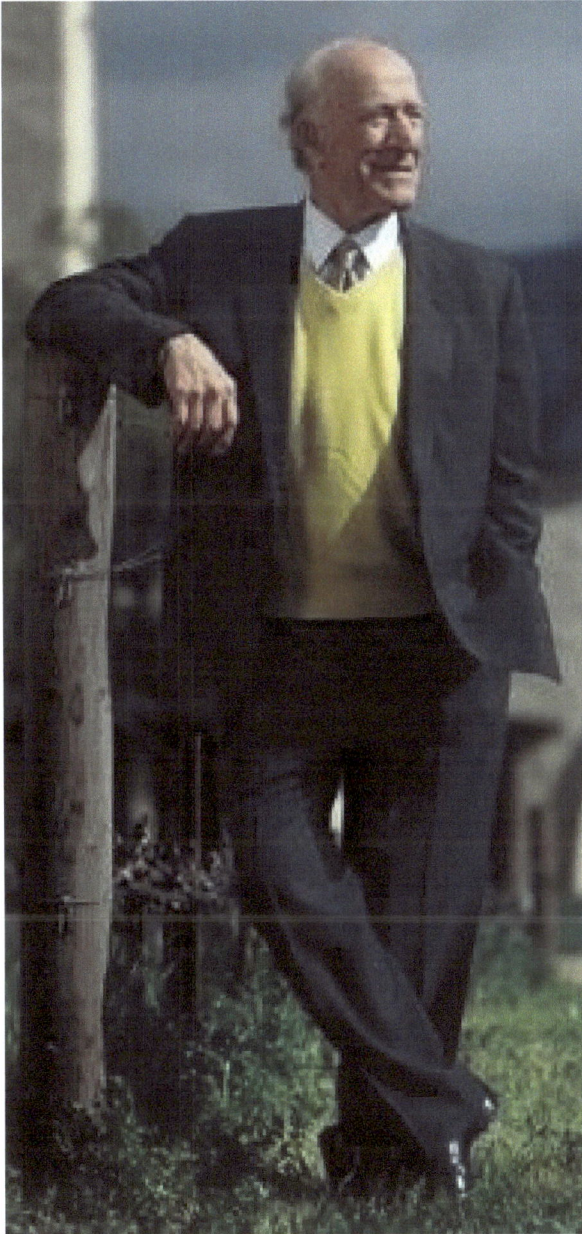

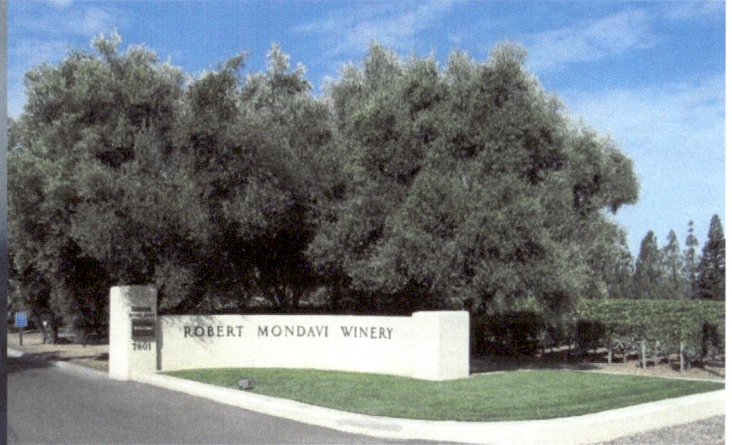

Born in Virginia, MN, to parents who emigrated from Italy, Robert Mondavi was greatly influenced by Old World traditions of the pleasures of wine and food. The family moved to Lodi, California, during Prohibition times attending public schools there. A 1936 graduate of Stanford University with a degree in economics and business administration, Robert understood that marketing was critical in achieving success in the wine industry. He joined his father at Sunnyhill Winery in Santa Helena, but, after convincing him to purchase the pioneering Charles Krug Winery there, he upgraded the technology determined to raise quality, a commitment which never faltered.

At 53, with little money but full of energy and vision, Robert Mondavi changed the course of the United States wine industry. Realizing his long-held dream to create excellent wines in the Napa Valley that would stand in the company of the great wines of the world, he founded the iconic Robert Mondavi Winery in 1966, opening the door to the future of American fine wine.

Robert knew that the first place to begin was in the vineyard. For the home of his winery he choose a 12 acres site in the "To Kalon" Vineyard (Greek for "the beautiful"). Its optimum sun exposure, an annual rainfall combined with a well-drained, gravelly clay soils contributes to the Napa Valley typical outstanding quality of the grapes. "As I walked the property, admiring its contours and vines, smelling the richness of its soil, I knew it was a very special place. The feeling was almost mystical" cited Robert.

He ordered to design the winery as an homage to California's early missions. The warm earth-toned arms of the building soon embraced visitors for wine tastings, tours and cultural programs – common activities at many wineries today but a radical idea at the time – letting them also enjoy great collections of sculptures and antiquities assembled by Robert and his wife, Margrit Biever Mondavi.

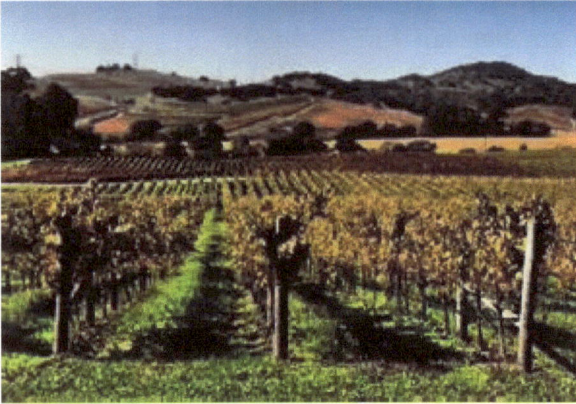

Over the years, more parcels of the historic To Kalon property alone have been adquired; the vineyard now stands at 550 acres featuring other innovations, such as gentle winemaking techniques that increase wine quality and natural farming practices that protect people and the environment, leading to fundamental changes in the industry's approach to winegrowing. "We were hearing all about it over in France, everyone was talking" remembers Genevieve Janssens, current Director of Winemaking, first working at the Robert Mondavi Winery in 1977. Two years later "Opus One", Mondavi's masterpiece in association with Baron Phillipe de Rothschild, was launched in the international market becoming a "classic Meritage blend".

To fulfill his vision of putting great wines on every table, Robert Mondavi founded in 1979 Woodbridge Winery, near his boyhood home in Lodi, California, a region capable of producing quality wines of exceptional value, raising this way the standard for everyday wine consumption.

Been California alone the fourth largest wine producer in the world, the Robert Mondavi Winery is today, without a doubt, the top fine wine producer in America. Describing and highly recommending its last releases:

Fumé Blanc Reserve 2009. To Kalon Vineyard (98% Sauvignon Blanc – 2% Semillon): Magnolia and verbena flowers open to lemon and grapefruit aromas with a hint of ginger and cardamom. Flavors of fresh nectarine are carried by a round, ample mouthfeel which finishes with light citrus.

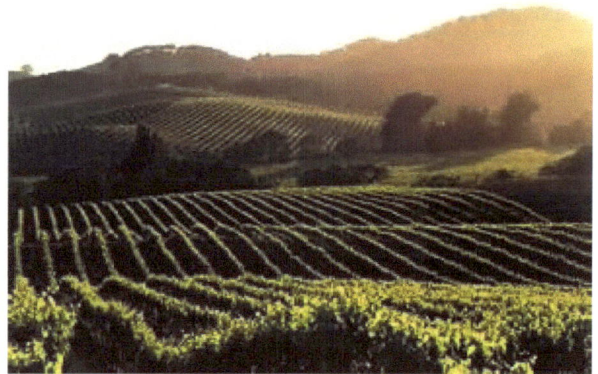

Fumé Blanc 2088. Napa Valley (98% Sauvignon Blanc – 2% Semillon): Intense primary aromas of lemongrass mingle with subtle scent of lime blossoms and hints of sage and spice. Mouthfilling flavors of crisp yellow peach are couched in a very smooth, rounded texture. Thanks to the small Semillon Blanc yields of 2008, flavors are concentrated and the vine is already very expressive in its youth. Both wines are excellent accompanying seafood and fresh fruits.

Chardonnay 2009. Private Section (96% Chardonnay – 2% Gewurtztraminer – 2% Riesling): The nose reveals lemon cream, orange zest and peach aromas with smoky oak nuances and enticing vanilla/brown sugar scents. The creamy, mouth-filling palate creates a lush impression and is balanced by a long crisp finish. Enjoy this delicious wine with rich seafood, poultry and pork dishes, white sauce pastas or soft-ripening cheeses.

Meritage 2009. Private Selection (41% Merlot – 35% Cabernet Sauvignon – 11% Petit Verdot – 10% Malbec – 3% Cabernet Franc): Inspired by Robert Mondavi's European travels, this Meritage blend is rich and potent, yet elegant and complex. It is a collage of the classic Bordeaux red varieties. In the glass, it offers lavish dark plum, black cherry and blackberry aromas along with a velvety texture and succulent mid-palate flavors.

Its finish is impressively long and enhanced by well integrated tannins. A superb match for hearty, richly lavored foods such as grilled steaks, lamb chops, osso bucco and flavorful cheeses.

Cabernet Sauvignon Reserve. Napa Valley (90% Cabernet Sauvignon – 7% Cabernet Franc – 3% Petit Verdot) Full, classic aromas of crème de cassis, licorice and cedarwood with layers of spice, camphor and roasted herbs.
On the palate, expressions of the To Kalon *terroir* manifest in ripe mineral-laced blue and black fruits wrapped in firm, velvety tannins and followed by an exceedingly long, aristocratic finish. Ideal with all red meats, game and aromatic cheeses.

Woodbridge Moscato 2010 (94.4% Muscat Alexander – 2.3% Chardonnay – 3.3% Aromatic white varietals) Easily identified by its intensely perfumed character, Muscat is believed to be the oldest known wine grape variety. The 2010 Moscato displays heady floral aromas of honeysuckle and rose accented on the palate with hints of orange zest and light lemon cream. The wine's lively acidity balances out the residual sugar and its slightly effervescent style makes it a delicious, stylish choice for many food pairings. Sip it in the afternoon with fruit and cheese or enjoy it with lightly sweet desserts. Serve chilled.

Woodbridge Brut Sparkling (100% Chardonnay): Perfect sparkling wine for celebrating the joy of everyday. Fresh citrus aromas are accented by soft, creamy yeast characters. Flavors of green apple and lemon cream linger along with the bubbles on the palate. *Robert Mondavi* believed that great wine was not just for special occasions. This new wine pairs well with a wide array of dishes, from shellfish appetizers to chicken entrées to luscious fruit desserts. It is also perfect on its own when a little celebrating is in order. Serve well chilled.

Robert Mondavi remained an active ambassador for the winery into his nineties, together with his wife, Magrit. He passed away peacefully at home at the age of 94.

Our eternal respect !

WINE AUCTIONS
A great investment in today's Financial World

In an era of stock market instability, declining real estate prices and little or no return for cash invested in money market or savings accounts, why not consider investing in wine? None of the existing documented records in wine history have ever registered a fall in market value. A bottle of a prestigious wine is also a great gift to a good friend. Reputable wine auctions can provide you with that opportunity, since, from a single bottle to numbered lots of large amount of cases, are available for bidding.

The product at the auctions come from anywhere and anyone – food & beverage operations, collectors, wine brokers, private clubs, inheritance recipients – in need of helpful cash. Even prestigious universities such as Oxford have been known to auction off parts of their collections. Most sellers remain anonymous, unless their names add some cachet, such the recent sale of rare Cognacs from the estate of American heiress Doris Duke at Chritie's of London. Auctions houses hold lavish tasting events prior to the sale, often for a fee of less than $100.00. At the auction itself, aside from buying the sales catalogue, there is no financial obligation. Winners pay what they bid, plus a buyer's commission of 10% to 20%. Catalogues are packed with most relevant information about provenance – the lineage of the wine – storage and condition. Where the wine has been since it left the *Chateau;* whether it has been in an appropriate humidity and temperature-controlled environment and, above all, the condition of the labels, closures and the all-important *ullage*, the space or "nobody's land" appearing between the surface of the wine and the cap. A certain amount of liquid is bound to evaporate over time, but too much air may indicate a problem with the cork or that the bottle was improperly filled. All these details are of vital importance when the buyer is involved in thousands of dollars transactions. Wine auction are fun, dynamic events with many different sorts of attendees.

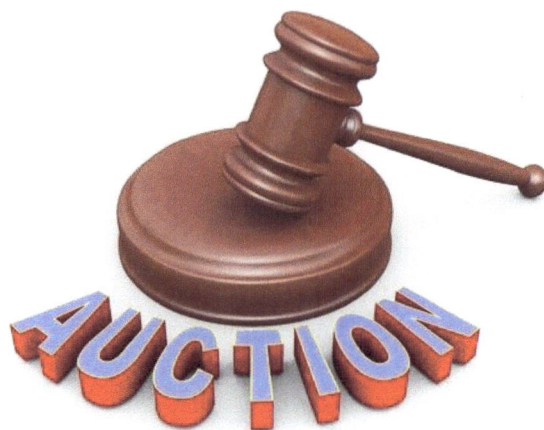

The audience typically ranges from hard core, cagey veterans to novices exploring the world of wine investment for the first time, along with everyone in between.

When looking to seriously invest in wine we recommend as a first step consulting the *Wine Market Journal*, publisher of the *Top 500* list of the world's all-time highly collectible wines from France, Italy, America, Spain and Portugal. In most cases the wines of Bordeaux are the highest value carriers in auctions, reason why a thoughtful analysis is needed, paying particular attention to the **1855 Classification of the Wines of Gironde**. This historical document, commissioned by the Emperor Napoleon III, categorizes the wines of the Medoc region into a five-tiered hierarchy deemed **First Growths** – Lafite, Latour, Haut Brion, Margaux, Mouton – showing some of the highest rates of return in terms of investment. France's Burgundy region is a bit more difficult to navigate but, when in doubt, just remember three letters: **DRC** – Domaine de la Romanée-Conti – . This impeccably managed estate has performed consistently well, with record high prices for their stable of wines that includes Romanée-Conti, La Tache, Richebourg, Romané St. Vivant, Grand Echézaux, Echézaux and Le Montrachet. Italy and Spain tend to play more of a supporting role in the auction/investment arena. Names worth pursuing would be Gaja and Bruno Giacosa for Italy and Vega Sicilia in Spain. Investors in California wines, Napa in particular, should be aware of the enormous appeal of such favorites as Harlam, Screaming Eagle, Colgin, Bryant Family and Scarecrow. These micro-production wineries have been generating strong numbers over the past year or two. **rep**

Most utable auction houses, such as Sotheby's, Christie's and Hart-Davis, have offered rare and outstanding vintage wines for many years to collectors and aficionados.Launched in 2009, **SPECTRUM WINE AUCTIONS**, a subsidiary of Spectrum Group International, a *Fortune 500* company, is the newest live and online auction house of fine collectible wines. As a vivid example of their successful accomplishments let's analyze the following results of its last Spring Auctions held in Costa Mesa (California) and Hong Kong. These are the top 10 lots sold:

1 – 12 Bottles of 1978 **DRC.** Domaine de la Romanée-Conti at $143,400
2 – 1 Imperial (6 Litters) of 2005 **DRC.** La Tache at $50,787
3 – 3 Magnums (1.5 Lt.) of 2005 **DRC.** Romanée-Conti at $83,650
4 – 3 Bottles of 1978 **DRC Henry Jayer.** Richebourg at $29,278
5 – 1 Jeroboam (4.5 Lt.) of 1982 Chateau Lafite Rothschild at 22,845
6 – 1 Bottle of 1945 Chateau Petrus, Pomerol, Grand Cru Classé at $6,573
7 – 1 Nabuccodonosor (15 Lt.) of 2005 Chateau d'Yquem at 14,340
8 – 12 Bottles of 1982 Chateau Lafite Rothschild at $47,800
9 – 12 Bottles of 1982 Chateau Mouton Rothschild in 3 separate lots for a total of $49,593
10 –60 Bottles in 3 separate lots of 20. 1995-1998 of Screaming Eagle Cabernet Sauvignon (Napa).

Total $85,443

All wines carry an insurance policy that covers its value while it is in transit as well as once it is in the buyer's possession. Bidding online gives the prospective buyers the opportunity to participate from the comfort of their own homes and also to bid on various auctions at once.

All potential investors, buyers and sellers alike, will find through these auctions the most accessible and expansive means and opportunities of enjoying what is simply the greatest consumable and collectible product known to man: Wine.

A VITICULTURAL GLORY OF SPAIN

The saga of the Codorníu Raventós family

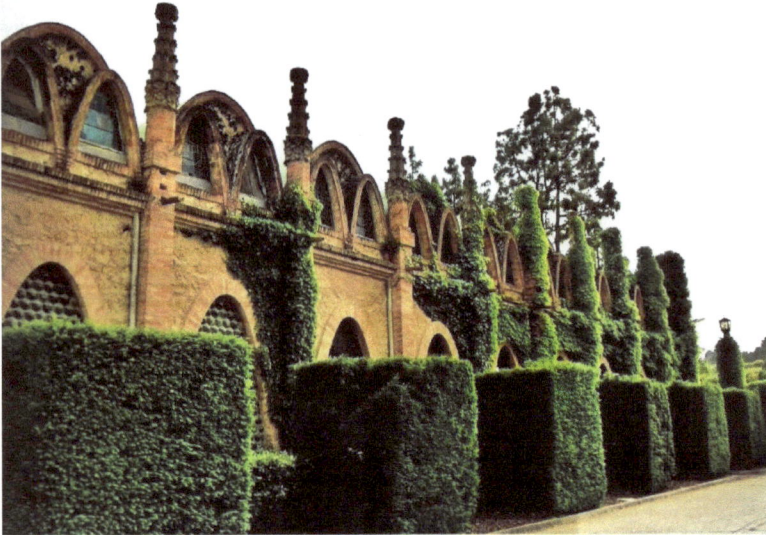

One of Spain's first wine families, Codorníu has been growing grapes in the *Cataluña* region since 1551. A document from that year shows that Jaume Codorníu owned vineyards and was operating a winery in San Sadurní, outside of Barcelona. In 1659, Anna de Codorníu and Miquel Raventós married, bringing the two winemaking families together and creating the foundations for the winery as we know it today. From the very first bottle, the Codorníu Raventós family revolutionized the Spanish wine industry expanding their production into the most important regions of Spain, including Rioja, Ribera del Duero and Priorat – in addition to global ownership of Artesa in Napa Valley and Bodega Séptima in Argentina. The Codorníu Raventós portfolio includes a selection of top quality Spanish wineries that capture the rich winemaking tradition of Spain and the spirit of innovation that has made the family-owned company a respected world leader in viticulture and winemaking.

With a production of more than 25 wines and spirits, we are presenting this illustrious *Bodegas* and their "stars":

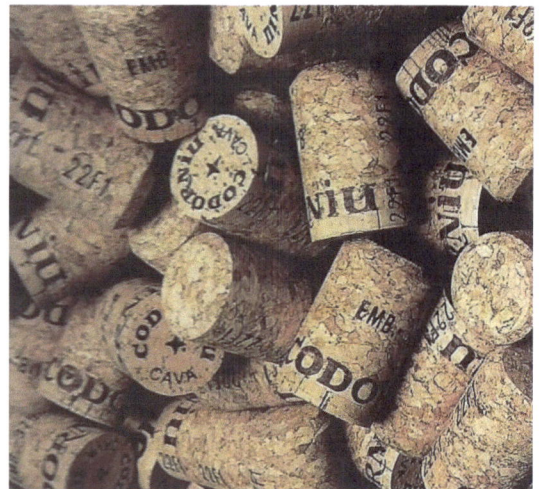

BODEGAS BILBAINAS – Viña Pomal 2006 Gran Reserva (90% Tempranillo – 10% Graciano) : A Rioja classic since 1911, first planted in 1908..The 2006 vintage was rated "Very Good" by most wine critics. It required considerable work in the vineyard. Rainfall was abundant which led to a great vegetative growth. Continuous monitoring was required, including extensive pruning to keep the vines stable. The wine is racked and clarified before being placed in American oak barrels for 24 months, spending a year in oak vats and 3 years in bottle prior to release. An impressive Red ideal for grilled meats and all cheeses. Alcohol content: 14%.

"SCALA DEI"– Garnatxa 2013 (100% Garnacha): The 2013 was a complex vintage to manage. It did not rain throughout the whole summer and the harvest ended one week earlier than usual. These drought conditions yielded very good quality on the more vigorous vineyards. In the end these wines present highly concentrated fruit and aromas. A young smooth red wine recommended with veal, poultry, pastas and soft cheeses. Alcohol content: 14%.

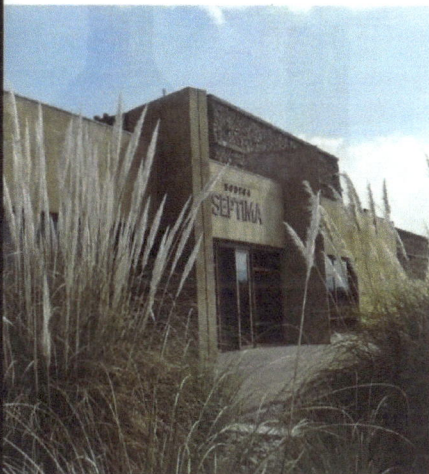

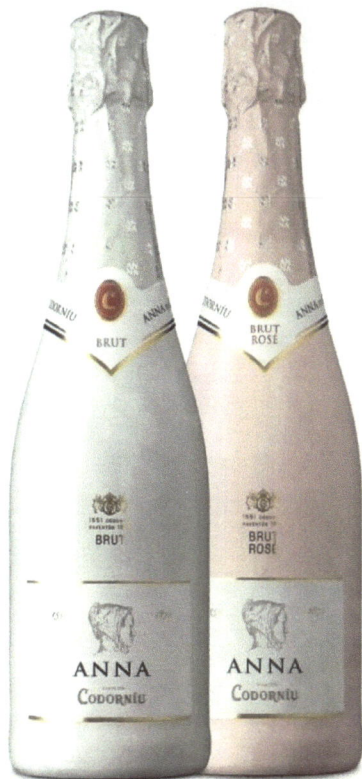

LEGARIS – Verdejo 2013 (100% Verdejo): This wine was born in 2009, marking the winery's first introduction to white varieties in the acclaimed region of Rueda. At an altitude of 2,300 – 2,700 feet above the sea level. Traditionally grown in bush vines, in recent years all the new plantation have adopted trellised vines which are mechanically harvested by night and the bush vines were harvested by hand during the day. Once the grapes were destemed and lightly crush, the wine then racked and left on its lees for at least two months. It did not undergo malolactic fermentation or aging in barrels. After final clarification, cold stabilization and filtering the wine ensured optimum stability, smoothness and presentation. Great with fresh fish and seafood, fruit salads and oriental dishes. Alcohol content: 12%.

ANNA DE CODORNIU – Cava Brut (70% Chardonnay – 30% Parellada): Cava is the typical sparkling wine that undergoes the *Métode Champanoise* in its elaboration influenced by the *Champagne* from the neighboring France. The grapes used in the production of Anna de Codorníu are sourced from two different growing areas. The Chardonnay grapes come from Lleida in the Cava region and the Parellada variety proceeds from the vineyards in the Penedés area. The zones hot Mediterranean climate allows for early fruit ripening and guarantees a good level of acidity and freshness accompanied by citrus and floral aromas. Fantastic wine for celebrations and, practically, most elegant cuisine and desserts. Alcohol content: 11.5%.

ANNA DE CODORNIU – Cava Brut Rosé (70% Pinot Noir – 30% Chardonnay): This is the sister wine to Codorníu' most iconic sparkling wine. Both the Pinot Noir and Chardonnay grapes come from vineyards located in Lleida, known for a continental climate that provides the grapes with optimum concentration, lower acidity and greater body and intensity. After harvest, taking place towards the middle of August and carried out at night, the Chardonnay grapes are destemed and pressed and the Pinot Noir must is left in contact with the skins for three or four hours to achieved its pink color. Once their fermentation is complete and the wines have been clarified, blending takes place and the resulting wine is bottled. The bottles are stored in underground cellars where a second fermentation occurs followed by a period of at least 12 months in cellar, until which the bottles are disgorged.

Finally, the definitive cork is inserted in the bottle. This wine is equally recommended with the same type of cuisine than the Cava Brut.

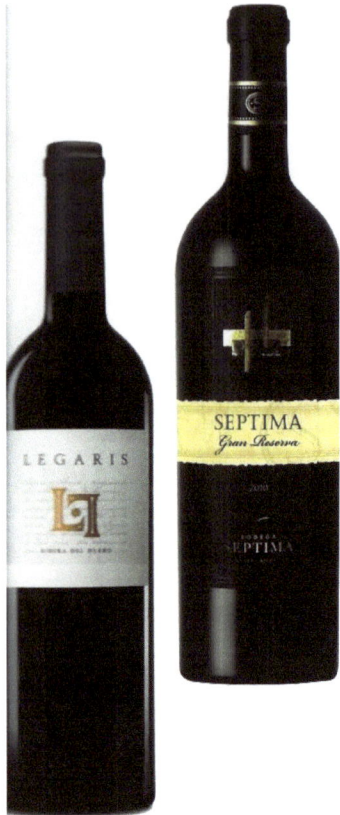

SEPTIMA Gran Reserva 2010 (55% Malbec – 30% Cabernet Sauvignon – 15% Tannat):

The wine was made with grapes grown in the Mendoza River and Uco Valley (Argentina) from three vineyards planted between 2,800 and 3,600 feet above sea level. The three wines that were blended for this Gran Reserva aged separately in French and American oak barrels for about 12 months. The color is deep purple with violet hues. The aromas are complex and expressive with the right level of toasts and subtle aromas of violets, dark chocolate and strawberry jam. The palate is elegant and balanced. The warm, sweet impact with marked tannins offers great volume in the mid-palate and overall balanced oak with mature red fruit end in a lingering finish. Great to accompany red meats, pastas, spicy dishes and all cheeses. Alcohol content 14.5%.

ARTESA Carneros Chardonnay 2012 (100% Chardonnay): The Chardonnay vineyards span the entire cool climate of the Carneros region in California. This wine is first and foremost about aromatics, and the techniques used are designed to retain the typical Carneros aromas of lemon-citrus and white blossom, while accentuating the minerality and vivid, fresh fruit flavors. Recommended with fresh fish and seafood, poultry, fruits and vegetarian dishes. Alcohol content 15.2%

"Thank you, Codorníu Dinasty" !

THE MAGIC OF CHAMPAGNE "TAITTINGER"

Worldwide recognized among connoisseurs and wine lovers

"**Taittinger**" is one of the remaining family owned and operated Champagne Houses.

The firm is distinguished for its extensive vineyards holdings of 752 acres, including prestigious Grand Cru vineyards in the Cotes des Blancs and Montagne de Reims regions. Unlike most houses, Champagne Taittinger relies primarily on estate grown grapes for its production.

Also unique are the higher proportion of

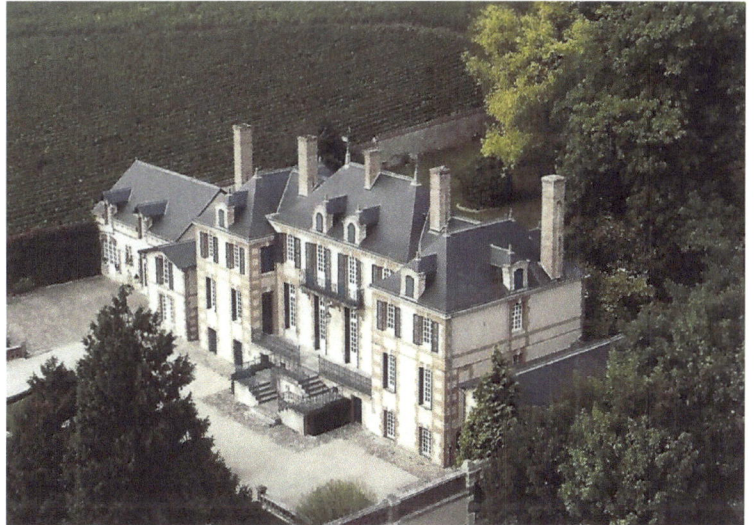

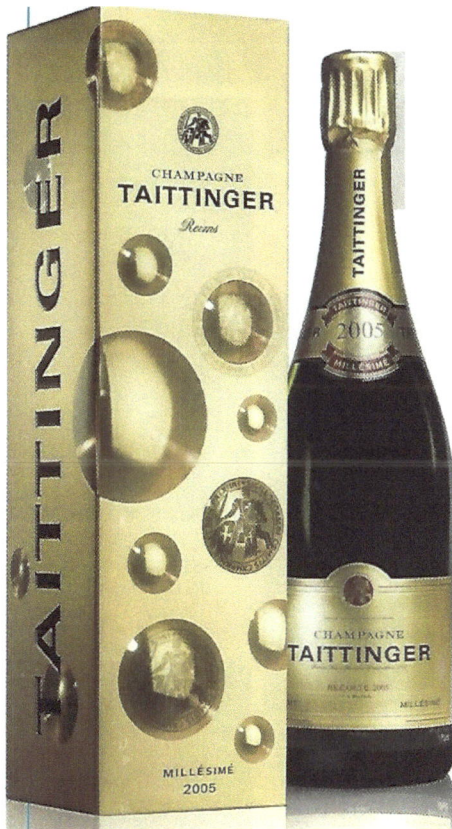

Chardonnay variety in its wines that gives **"Taittinger"** its signature style, and the time devoted to aging the wines before release – most often greatly exceeding the official requirement – in a practice that also has become a "Taittinger" hallmark.

The House of Taittinger was founded upon a promise that Pierre Taittinger made to himself in 1915 when he was a young cavalry officer serving in the First World War, with his company headquarters at the Chateau de la Marquetterie, two mile from Epernay, near the Marne river. Captivated by the lovely 18th-century residence, the young Taittinger was determined to purchase it, should the opportunity arise. By September 1930 he had adquired the venerable Champagne firm of Forest-Fourneaux, founded in 1734 and the third oldest Champagne House in existence at the time. Two years later, after restructuring the firm and expanding its vineyards holdings, Pierre Taittinger kept his promise of purchasing the Chateau de la Marquetterie and its surrounding vineyards – as well as the Comptes de Champagne residence in downtown Reims. Pierre, as a master of the culinary arts, created a visionary evolution centered on two concepts: lightness and naturalness. This standards continued uninterrupted until today.

These are the jewels of "Taittiger" extensive collection, soul of all celebrations:

BRUT LA FRANCAISE_N.V.(40% Chardonnay, 35% Pinot Noir, 25% Pinot Meunier):

The presses are located in the vineyard for immediate pressing of the fruit. The resulting must is resting until the end of winter, to follow undergoing a second fermentation in the bottle for almost 4 years, allowing the wine to reach the pick of aromatic maturity. The result, is a delicately balanced champagne. This wine has a subtle, pale gold color with fine, persistent bubbles. With aromas of peach, white flowers, vanilla pod and brioche, presents flavors of fresh fruits and honey on the palate. Excellent as an aperitif or foods such as fresh seafood, fowl and white meats.

Pierre-Emmanuel Taittinger, grandson of the founder, with daughter Vitalie and son Clovis

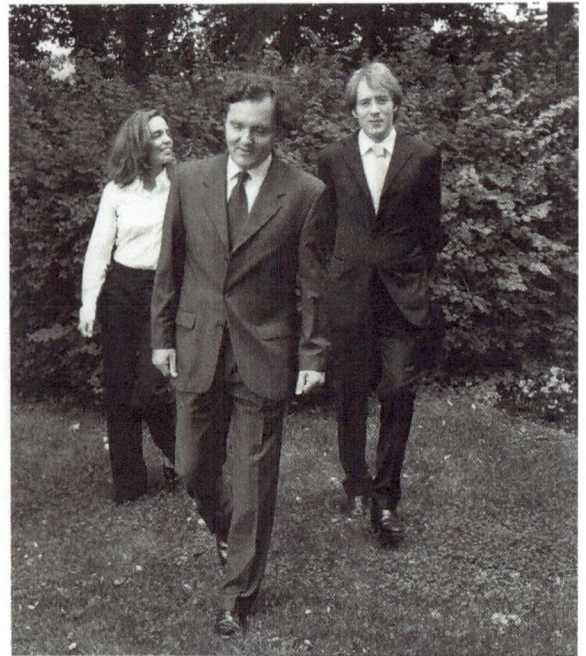

COMPTES DE CHAMPAGNE BLANC DE BLANCS (100% Chardonnay): Produced only in exceptional vintage years and intended as the ultimate expression of the Taittinger style, this wine is composed entirely of Chardonnay grapes grown in the top vineyards of the prestigious Cotes des Blancs. Only the first press juice is used. A small proportion (5%) of the blend spends three to four months in new oak barrels, enhancing the intrinsic qualitiesof the final blend. Prior to disgorgement, the Blanc de Blancs is aged for 10 years on the lees in the 13th-century chalk cellars that were once the property of Saint Nicaise Abbey.

A powerful, refined, expressive and complex Champagne, with notes of citrus fruits, lime blossom and caramelized grapefruit. The long, rich ending reveals sweet licorice aromas.

A perfect accompaniment to first courses such as seafood and shellfish. The greatest toast!

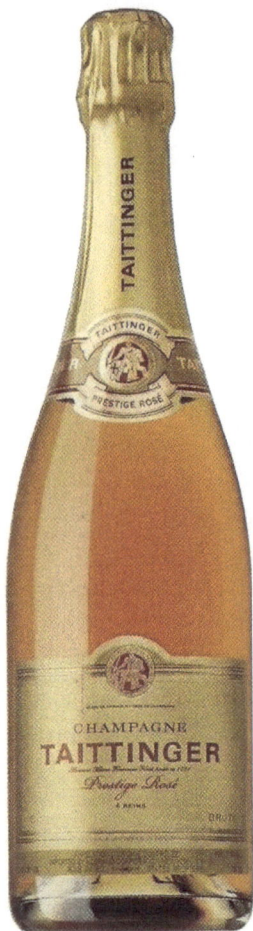

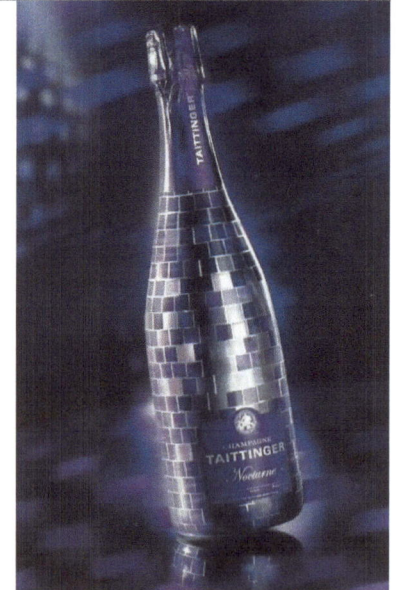

PRELUDE (50% Chardonnay, 50% Pinot Noir): This Champagne is produced exclusively From Grand Cru vineyards of Chardonnay from the Cotes des Blancs and plump grapes Pinot Noir from the Montagne de Reims. Pressed among the vineyards the must undergoes a second fermentation in the winery under temperature-controlled conditions in the bottle.

Under this process the wine acquires its complexity and fine, pinpoint bubbles. The wine is aged for five years to develop body and bouquet. The wine is pale yellow color with silvery reflections. Subtle and fresh on the nose, with mineral aromas that quickly give way to notes of elderflowers and spicy cinnamon. The lively palate is dominated by fresh citrus and white peaches in syrup giving way to a lingering finish that bursts with flavor. Makes an excellent aperitif or accompaniment to classic seafood dishes.

NOCTURNE (40% Chardonnay, 35% Pinot Noir, 25% Pinot Meunier): Recently added to this great collection. A blend of more than 35 different crus from a variety of harvests, this wine spends four years on the lees before being disgorged. A small dosage of cane sugar combined with the slow cellar aging creates a round, mellow, smooth Champagne that is perfect to enjoy with a dessert or late in the evening. This distinctive sweet Champagne is pale yellow in color with shimmering highlights and bubbles that form a delicate ring of fine foam. There are aromas of white flowers, yellow peach and dry apricots. The palate is smooth and creamy yet very crisp and gives way to flavors of raisins and fruit in syrup.

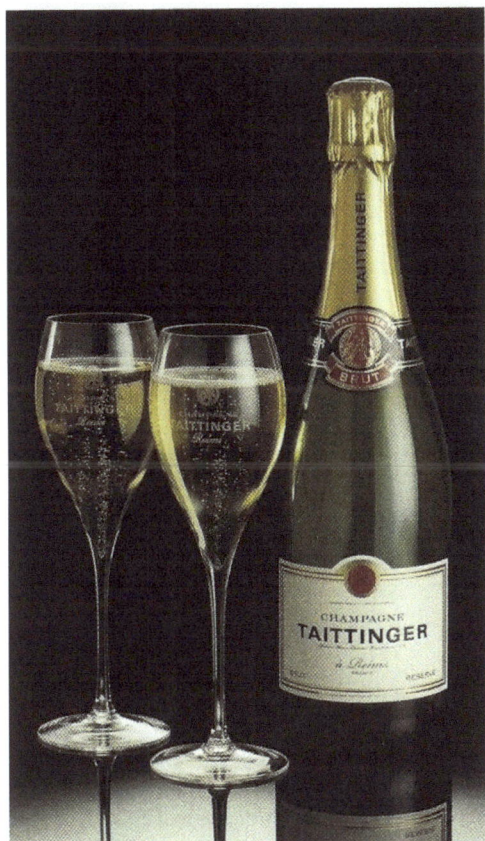

This mature, rich and round wine culminates in a long, smooth finish.

"Nocturne" is the perfect accompaniment to fruit desserts, lightly sweet pastry or cakes, as well as rich patés with toasted brioche.

PRESTIGE ROSE (50% Pinot Noir, 30% Chardonnay, 20% Pinot Meunier): Following the Taittinger style the majority of the fruit is pressed in the vineyards. At the winery the must undergoes a cool temperature fermentation. 85% of the blend is vinified as white wine and the reminder as red wine. The final cuvée is blended from an extensive range of at least 15 diverse crus of the Champagne region. After second fermentation in the bottle, the wine spends three years bottled to develop an extraordinary complexity and grandiose bouquet.

This cuvée presents a vibrant pink color with fine bubbles and persistent foam. The full and wonderfully expressive nose delivers aromas of crushed raspberries, cherries and black currants that lead into crisp, fresh red fruit flavors on the palate. Velvety and full-bodied, this wine is lively, fruity and fresh.

A delicious, fragrant aperitif, the wine is also subtle accompaniment to fruit desserts, including fruit tart, fruit salad and red fruit crumble.

Not bad for a wine that was discovered in the 16th-century by accident!

THE GREAT WINES OF PORTUGAL
ESPORAO Winery. Its worldwide Ambassador

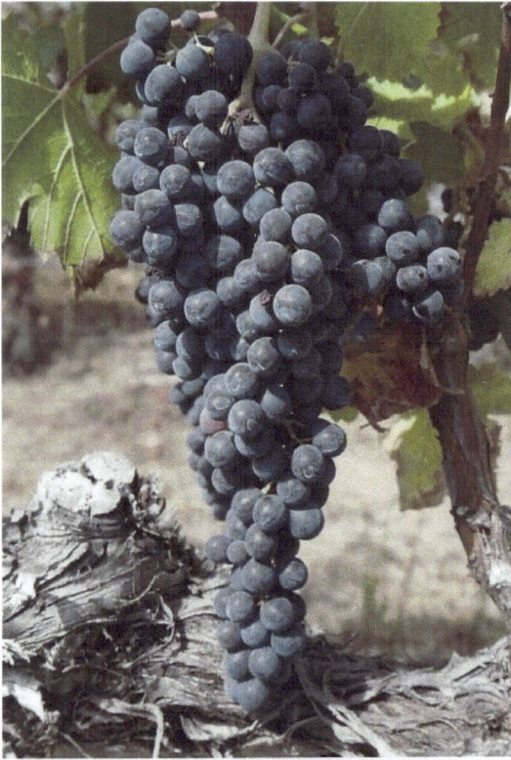

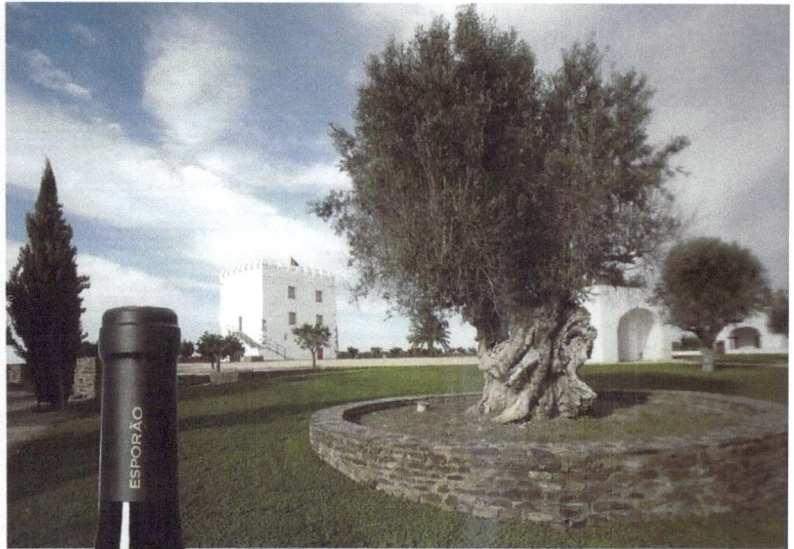

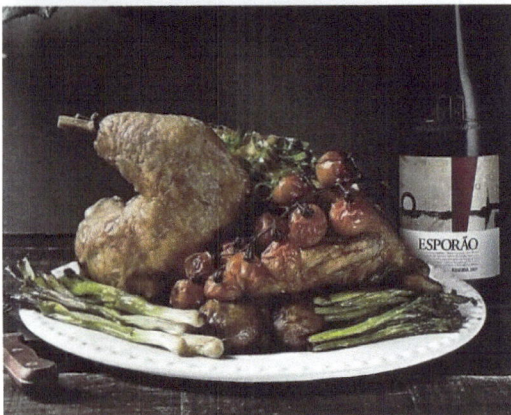

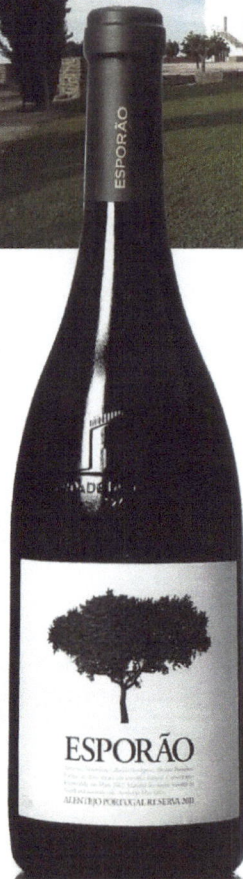

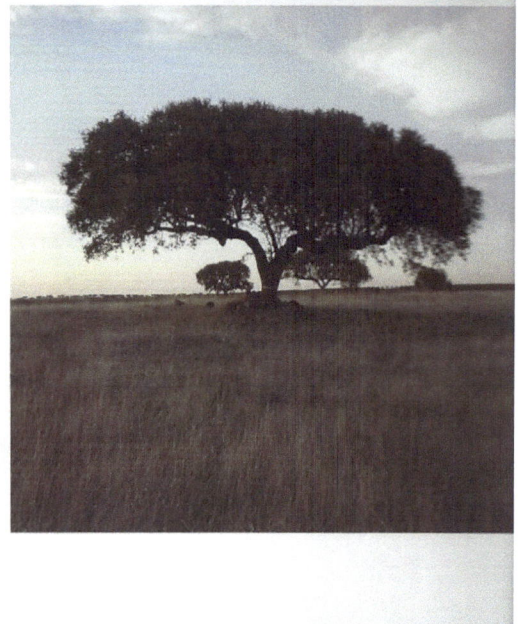

In the remote Alentejo region, 112 miles east of Lisbon, the ESPORAO estate seems indifferent to the pace of time. The largest and oldest fortification of the region stretches out to boundaries that were established as far back as 1267 and they pride themselves on growing local traditional grape varieties dating back to Roman Times. The vineyards and olive groves of the state stretch over 3,700 acres and benefit from exceptional conditions of climate, geology and irrigation.

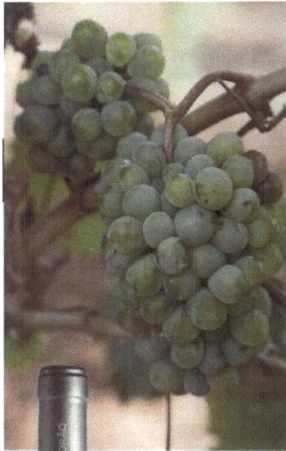

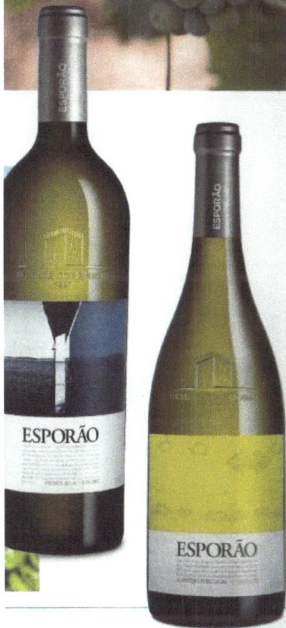

The generosity of the Douro river and volcanic soils produce sparkling, fortified and table wines made from the finest grape varieties, mostly of Portuguese origin. The different characteristics of the wines are honed under an intense sun, tempered by a humid Atlantic breeze. Since its creation," Esporao" wines has always been acutely concern with pre-serving the environment and nature. This concern is reflected in the company's philosophy and all who work with it. "Esporao" is committed to defining best practices for wine, olive growing and forestry with the aim of encouraging bio-diversity and minimizing soil erosion. Also the culture of a wide range of original genetic grape varieties is encouraged as well as minimal use of pesticides in the vineyards, aiming for a sustained and natural environment for grape growing. The two large wine producing properties are HERDADE DO ESPORAO and QUINTA DOS MURCAS. We are presenting the excellence of their most recently released wines:

Esporao :

Private Selection White 2012 – (100% Semillon):Color: Crystal clear, straw with green tinges. Aroma: Ripe citric and tropical fruit aromatics, combining with complex white chocolate and toasty oak notes. Palate: Well balanced palate which is both elegant and unctuous. Long and persistent finish.

White Reserve 2013 – (Antao Vaz, Arinto, Roupeiro, Semillon): Color: Clear, straw with green tinges. Aroma: Rich, intense, notes of peach and grapefruit, well integrated toasty notes. Palate: Creamy and complex, well balanced, deeply fruity with minerality and a fresh persistent finish.

Private Selection Red 2009 – (Alicante Bouschet, Aragonés, Syrah): Color: Deep dense red. Aroma: Rich aromas of ripe red berry fruits with smokey tones. Palate: Intense, compact palate with firm tannins, well structure, finishing long and with good persistence.

Red Reserve 2011- (Aragonés, Trincadeira, Cabernet Sauvignon and Alicante Bouschet): Color: Deep dark red . Aroma: Intense spicy, dense and creamy. Firm tannins offering structure for bottle maturation.

Qinta dos Murcas:

Red Reserve 2009 – (Tinta Roriz, Tinta Amarela, Tinta Barroca, Touriga Nacional Touriga Francesa, Sousao). Color: Dense, almost opaque with purple edges. Aroma: Mature blue and blackberry fruit with subtle dark chocolate notes. Palate: Opulent and compact with elegant fruit notes and subtle oak. Well balanced and structured for bottle ageing.

Enjoy this centuries old excellence Salud !

"RIBERA DEL DUERO"
The pinnacle of Spanish winemaking from the lands of Castilla

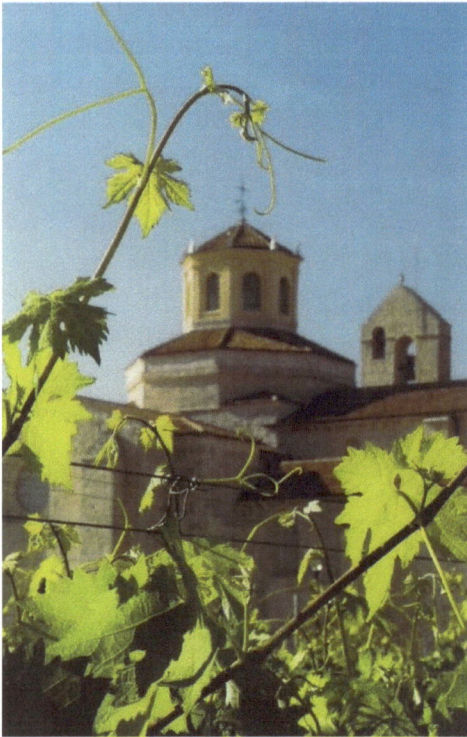

Located in Spain's northern plateau approximately two hours directly north of Madrid, Ribera del Duero extends over parts of four provinces of Castilla: Burgos – with the highest yielding vineyards – Segovia, Soria and Valladolid, where we can find most of the wineries. Ribera, which means "river bank", is defined in geophric terms by the horizontal axis of the Duero River, crossing central Spain from east to west. Enjoying a Mediterranean climate with Continental influences, the region ensures ideal conditions for the production of great quality wines.

Officially, the Denomination de Origen (D.O.) of Ribera del Duero was founded in 1982 by an organization of wine producers and growers who were determined to promote the quality of their wines and enforce regulatory standards.. In practice, winemaking in Ribera dates back over 2,000 years to the roman era, as evidenced by a recent find, a 66-meter mosaic of Bacchus, the god of wine, unearthed in the region.

In the middle ages, new plantings by Monastery monks such as Cistercians – first to arrive in the 12th Century – and the Benedictines from Cluny in Burgundy, spurred a revival in local winemaking. Ribera's earliest underground cellars with their distinctive chimneys were built in the 13th Century in towns across the region, and still serve today to protect wines from extreme climate. Ribera wines were highly regarded for export at the height of the Spanish Empire in the 17th and 18th centuries. Today, the newest technology and modern techniques as well as a respect for tradition have driven the quality of Ribera del Duero to its highest accomplishments in over two millennia of winemaking history. Its wines have received international acclaim and enjoy widespread distribution.

The main grape variety of the Ribera region is Tempranillo – of widespread cultivation in Spain –, which is locally known as Tinta del País or Tinto Fino. Tempranillo, an early-ripening variety, (from temprano"meaning "early"), is ideally suited to Ribera's short growing season due to climate's extreme conditions.

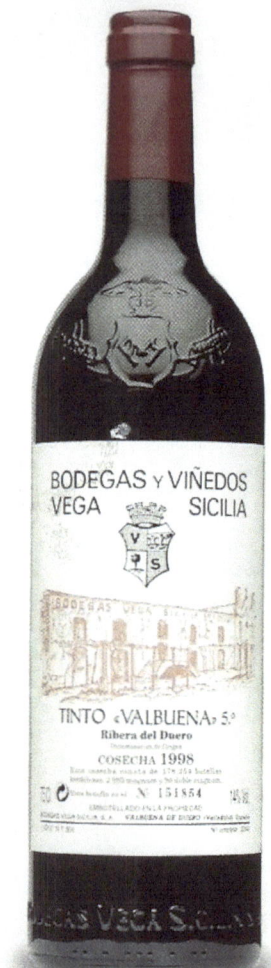

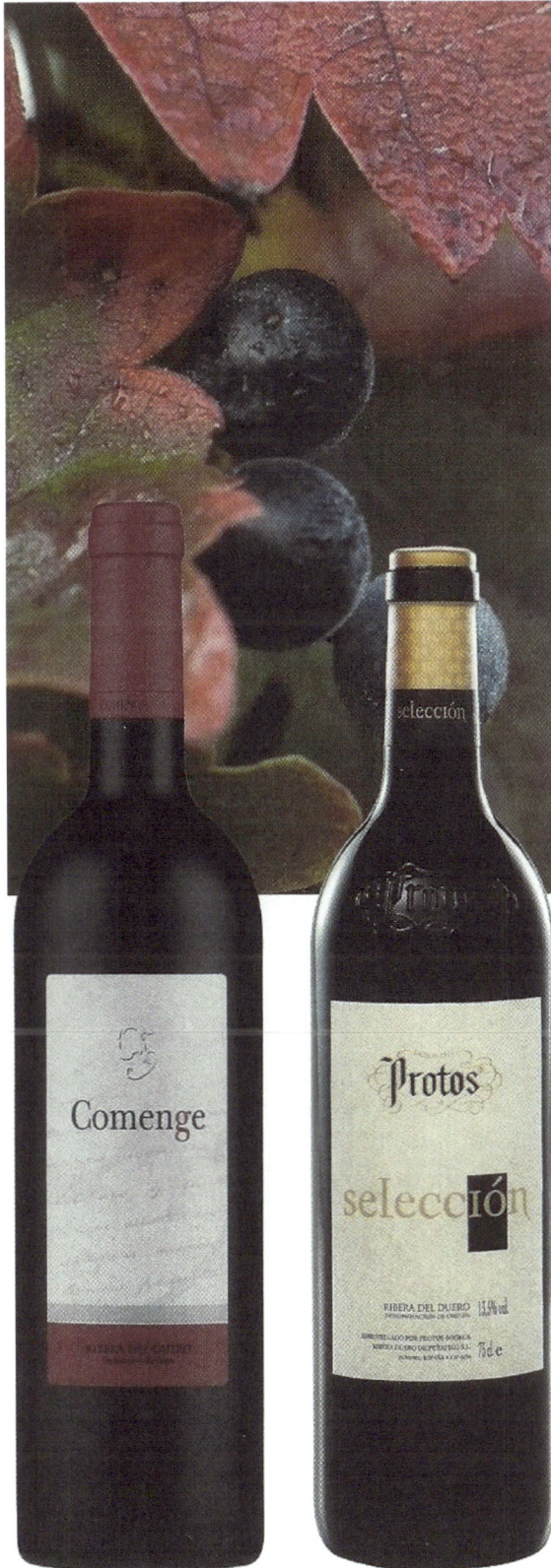

Apart from this main variety, Garnacha, Cabernet Sauvignon, Merlot, Malbec and the white variety Albillo are also cultivated. Many wine drinkers will wonder how Riberas differ from Riojas, if Tinta del País and Tempranillo are identical. In the Ribera region only a few wines are aged as long as traditional Riojas. Instead, they are marketed soon after fermentation in French and new American oak barrels.

Today there are well over 100 bodegas, with more springing up. The secret of this success lies in the region's red wines, which are exceptionally dark, superbly fruity, richly robust and remarkably well able to age if desired.

Among all the artisan Bodegas from **Ribera del Duero** we want to present the wines of the most prominent reputation:

VEGA SICILIA: Considered as the golden legend of Spanish red wine, has been the favorite to compliment the Royal Tables, High Dignitaries gatherings and top Corporate Covenants of the Old and New World.

The enterprise began in 1848 with the buying of 2,000-hectare estate from the Marquis de Valbuena and was 1915 the year marking the birth of two exceptional wines. Its distribution of these first bottles began among the upper class bourgeoisie and aristocracy, forging the legend of Spain's most exclusive wine, as it cannot be bough with money, but only with friendship. In today's market the Bodega excels with its *"top of the line"* VEGA SICILIA UNICO, which comes from the older vines on the estate blending a high percentage of Tempranillo with hints of Cabernet Sauvignon and Merlot. We also have to admire VEGA SICILIA COSECHA, VALBUENA "QUINTO ANO" and ALION a great popular selection.

PROTOS: Bodegas Protos was founded in 1927. The name Protos translate as "the first" in Greek. Its success is based on solid traditions combined with the best modern technology, from the 1.2 miles of corridors/cellars under the Peñafiel Castle – some dating from the middle ages – to the new building designed by Sir Richard Rogers.

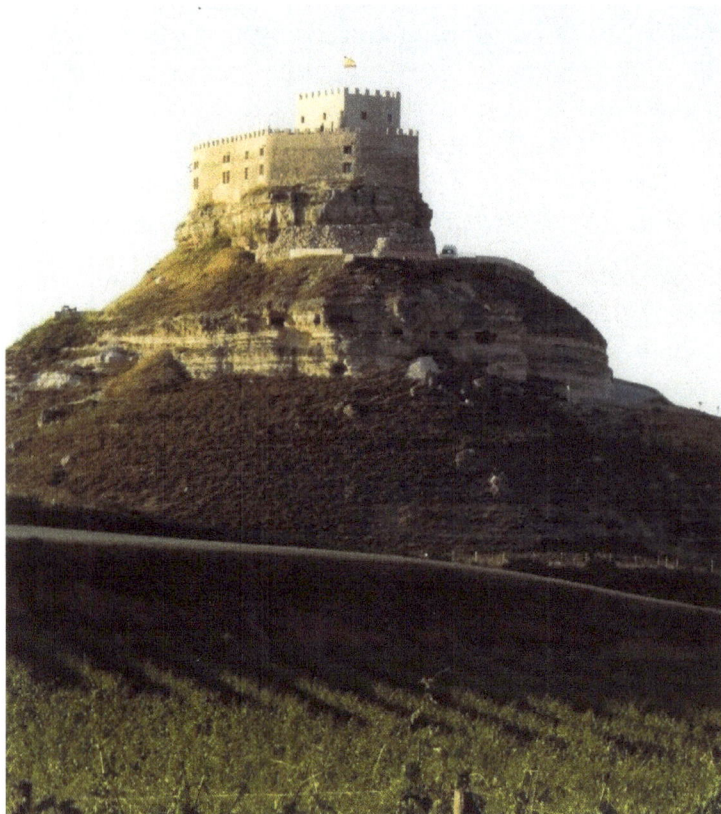

Their most celebrated wines are their CRIANZA, RESERVA, GRAN RESERVA and PROTOS SELECCION.

There also is a production of table wines of a great popularity: RIBERA DUERO and RIBERA DUERO TINTO.

From this collection emerges in excellence the PROTOS SELECTION: Ruby red color with violet rim. On the nose, this wine shows aromas of fruit well integrated with the oak. Vanilla and spices hints, toasts and liquorice coming through. On the palate, this wine has up-front fruit. It is powerful, well balanced, fleshy and luscious.

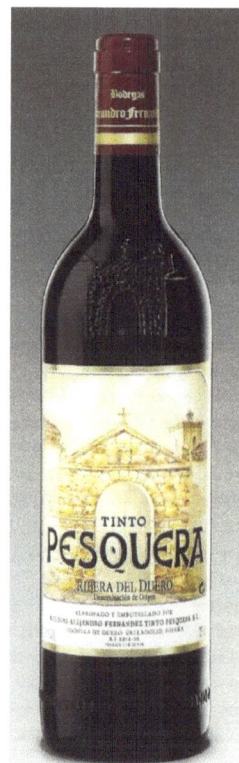

COMENGE: In order to honor his father, Don Miguel Comenge, Spain's illustrious oenologist and wine writer, his son Jaime Comenge founded the Bodega in 1999 sitting on a hillside with the Castle of Curiel on one side and the Castle of Peñafiel on the other. The views from the winery are nothing short of spectacular. The unique microclimate and soil allows a masterful cultivation of Tempranillo, which is the base for Comenge's magnificent and complex red wines, COMENGE CRIANZA and DON MIGUEL COMENGE RESERVA. Let's elaborate on this last one: Showing a splendorous deep cherry color in the glass, this Reserva offers an elegant bouquet with a wealth of fruit, truffles, tobacco and fine cocoa. In the palate it is round, tasty, well balanced, with smooth tannins and great elegance.

PESQUERA: Like many winemakers, Alejandro Fernández, Proprietor of Pesquera, pursued other careers before the dream of running his own bodega was realized. In 1972 Alejandro's dream began to take shape, as he and his wife, Esperanza, licensed their winery in the town of Pesquera in Ribera del Duero. The estate has now over 500 acres of mature vineyard , situated in a variety of soils. Vinification includes total destemming, maceration for up to twenty days an maturation in small oak barriques.

The wines are neither filtered nor cold-stabilized.

A real boutique-bodega. The Pesquera wine highlights are: RIBERA DEL DUERO CRIANZA, RIBERA DEL DUERO RESERVA 1997 y RIBERA DEL DUERO TINTO 1994. All wines with dense purple color. Aromas of berry fruit with delightful rich nuances of chocolate and spice and a nice creamy, very tannic finish.

Salud! From the land of El Cid.

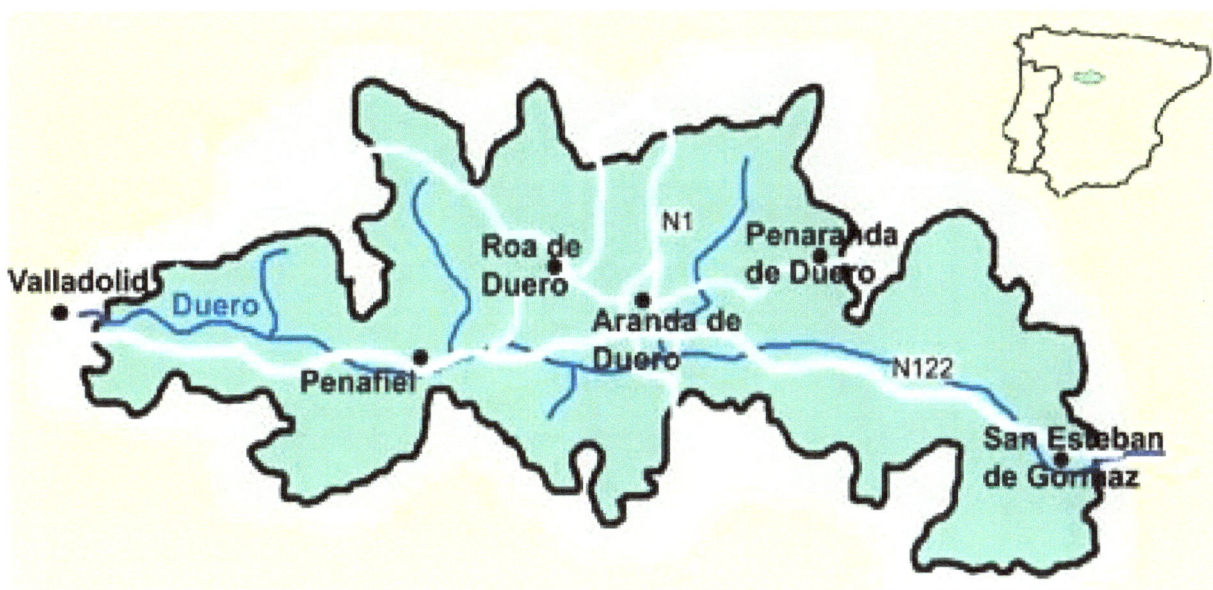

(Photos courtesy of Consejo Regulador. Ribera del Duero)

THE WINES OF CHILE
Nectar of The Americas

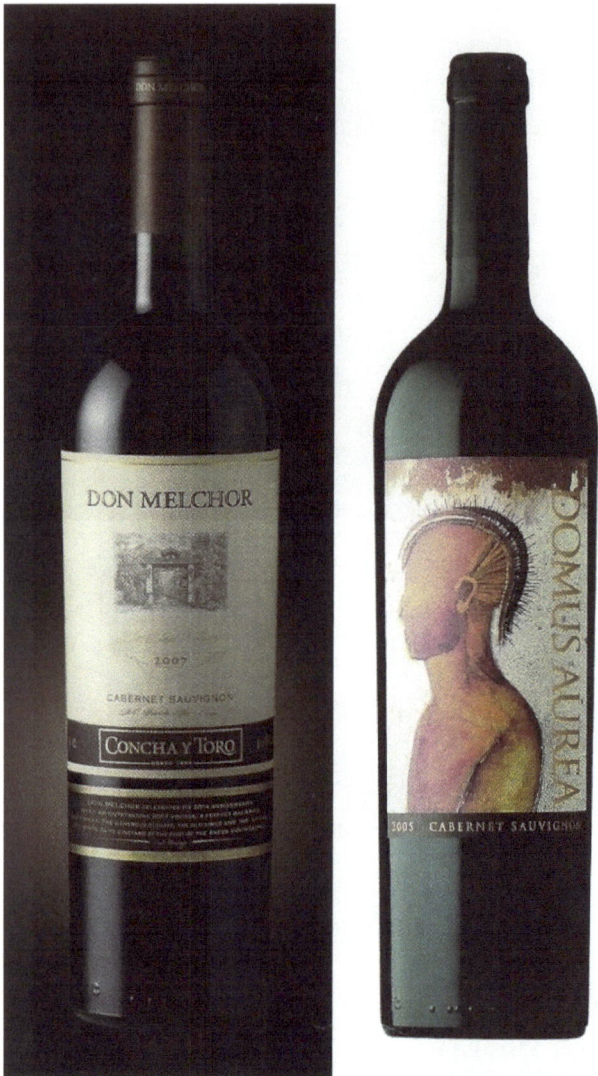

THE WINES OF CHILE

Chile is a long narrow country two times the size of California, that is geographically and climatically dominated by the Andes Mountains to the East, with a 3,000 miles of coastline from the Pacific Ocean to the West, the intense presence of the Atacama Desert in the North and the clima-severe Patagonia region to the South. ´

This diversity provoques a wide range of microclimates allowing to grow over twenty grape types in the country, mainly a mixture of French and Spanish varieties. To this day we find the cultivation of the reds Cabernet Sauvignon, Merlot, Carménere, Zinfandel, Pinot Noir, Petite Sirah, Cabernet Franc, Syrah, Sangiovese, Barbera, Malbec, Tempranillo, Pedro Ximénez and Cariñena. White wine varieties include Chardonnay, Sauvignon Blanc, Sauvignon Vert, Semillon, Riesling, Viognier, Torontel, Gewurztraminer and Muscat of Alexandría. Practically most European species are represented in this rich assortment, however, the grape that has become Chile's enological insignia, produced by most wineries and hold in the highest esteem in the industry is Carménere or *Grande Vidure*. A member of the Cabernet Sauvignon family, was originally planted in the Médoc region of Bordeaux, France, and used to produce deep red wines, occasionally for blending purposes.

European Vitis vinifera vines were brought to Chile by Spanish conquistadors and missionaries in the 16th century around 1554. Local legend states that the conquistador Francisco de Aguirre himself planted the first vines that, most likely, came from established Spanish vineyards planted in Peru which included the "common black grape", as it was known, that Hernán Cortés brought to Mexico in 1520. Jesuit priests cultivated this early vineyards using the wine for the celebration of the Eucharist. Despite being politically linked to Spain for centuries, Chilean wine history has been most profoundly influenced by the French, particularly the Bordeaux winemaking, due to the wealthy Chilean landowners visits to France.

By the beginning of the 19th century the imports of French vines to plant and contracting of oenologists to supervise the cultivation and winemaking techniques had a decisive surge in the country. The unfortunate entrance of *phylloxera* into the French vines turned into a positive event for the Chilean wine industry. Today Chile exports 68% of its wine production and is the third country in the U.S. wine imports list, after Italy and Australia.

The climate in Chile's wine regions is classified as Mediterranean, closely compared to California and Bordeaux, showing an average summer temperatures of 60 – 65 degrees Farenheit and potential highs of 85 degrees. In December 1994, the Republic of Chile defined the following viticultural regions:

Atacama: Comprising the Copiapó Valley and the Huasco Valley. The region is known primarily for its Pisco production and as a very important source of grape varieties.

Coquimbo: With 3 subregions, the Elqui, Limari and Choapa Valleys. Also important producers of Pisco and grape varieties.

Aconcagua: Within the Valparaiso province we'll find two of the greatest Chile's wine regions settled in the Aconcagua Valley, notable for its Cabernet Sauvignon and Merlot varieties and the Casablanca Valley well known for its Chardonnay and Pinot Noir wines.

Valle Central: The largest wine cultivation area which includes the Metropolitan Region. It spans the Maipo Valley, the Rapel Valley, the Curicó Valley and the Maule Valley. Their many microclimates and geological phenomena has triggered the employ of the latest advances in viticultural techniques to help vineyards in these areas compensate for some of these effects.

Southern Chile: Two sub regions are included, The Itata Valley and Bio-Bio Valley with high rainfall, lower average temperature and fewer hours of sunlight than the Northern Region.
Let's elaborate on the top Chile's wineries:

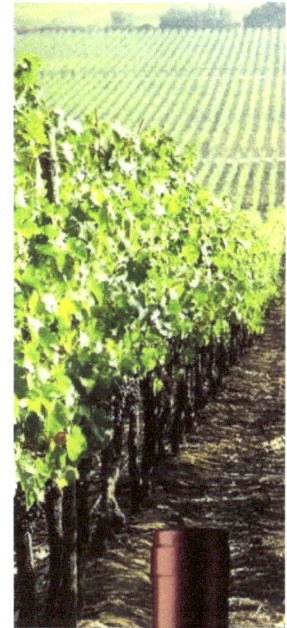

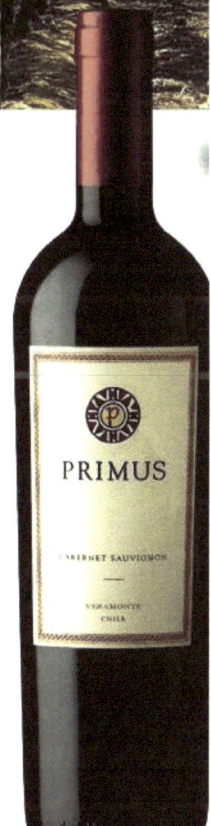

CASA LAPOSTOLLE (Casablanca): All vineyards are 100% managed organically and byodinamically. Their winemaking philosophy is based upon producing wines that express their unique *terroir* in total harmony with the environment. Most recent releases: CASA SAUVIGNON BLANC 2010 – CUVEE ALEXANDRE CHARDONNAY 2009 – CUVEE ALEXANDRE CARMENERE 2009 – CUVEE ALEXANDRE CABERNET SAUVIGNON 2009 – CLOS APALTA 2007.

VERAMONTE (Casablanca): The CasablancaValley climate is very similar to California's Russian River and the wines have power richness and depth with inky color. SAUVIGNON BLANC RESERVA 2010 – PINOT NOIR RESERVA 2009 – "PRIMUS" CABERNET SAUVIGNON 2008 – "PRIMUS" THE BLEND 2008.

SAN PEDRO (Maipo – Curicó): This winery masters their red blends to perfection. 1865 LIMITED EDITION (65% cabernet Sauvignon – 35% Syrah) – CABO DE HORNOS CABERNET SAUVIGNON 2006 (80% Cabernet Sauvignon – 15% Syrah – 5% Malbec).

COUSIÑO MACUL (Maipo): Over the years this winery has maintained its classic style by combining New World ripeness with Old World elegance. Last releases – SAUVIGNON GRIS 2009 – FINIS TERRAE 2007 (60% Cabernet Sauvignon – 40% Merlot) – ANTIGUAS RESERVAS 2007 (100% Cabernet Sauvignon).

CONCHA Y TORO (Maipo): The winery aims to be a leading global branded wine Company. With over a dozen different brands it is presently the largest winery in Chile. Stars of the collection: DON MELCHOR 2007 (100% Cabernet Sauvignon) A hearty assemblage of this varietal from different viticultural blocks. – ALMAVIVA "FIRST GROWTH" (100% Cabernet Sauvignon): This wine is a partnership between Cocha y Toro and Baron Philippe de Rothschild, owner of Chateau Mouton Rothschild in Bordeaux, in order to create a truly exceptional wine in the heart of the Maipo Valley.

MIGUEL TORRES (Curicó): The pioneer of the "New Wine" of Chile. His two masterpieces: CONDE DE SUPERUNDA: Blend of Cabernet Sauvignon, Carmenere, Monastrell and Tempranillo. Inspired in Don Miguel's Spanish tradition of winemaking. – MANSO DE VELASCO (100% Cabernet Sauvignon): Its name pays homage to the former Governor of Chile, famous for his strength in the battlefield and founder of Curicó.

The list of outstanding Chilean wineries is long and illustrious. We also want to mention the nobility of: **MONTES – KOYLE – DOMUS AUREA – CASA SILVA – SANTA RITA – VIÑA MAQUIS – APALTAGUA – KUYEN.**

Let's toast with the nectar of The Americas!

THE SINGLE MALT WHISKY
"The Dalmore" and "Jura". True expressions of Scotland

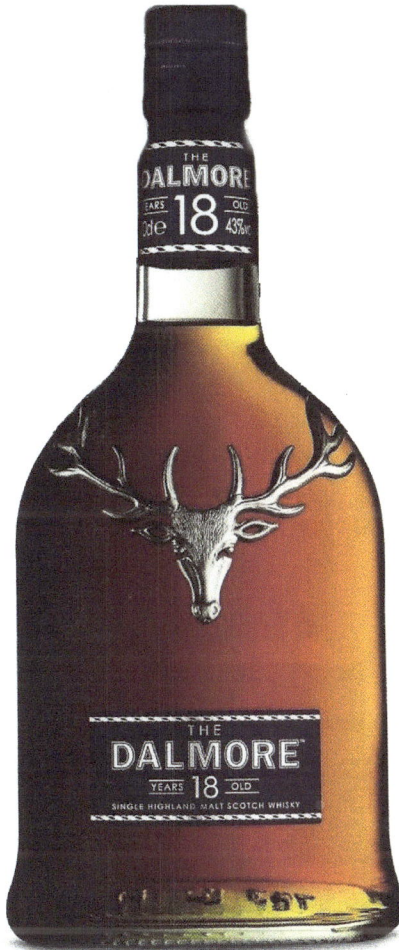

Distillation of whisky has been performed in Scotland for centuries. It is known the Celts distilled spirits from the beginning of time, however the earliest written record of whisky production in Scotland from malted barley is an entry on the 1494 Exchequer Rolls, which reads "Eight bolls of malt to Friar John Cor, by order of the King, wherewith to make aqua vitae". Single Malt Scotch is whisky made in Scotland using a pot still distillation process at a single distillery. As with any Scotch whisky, a Single Malt Scotch must be distilled in Scotland and matured in oak casks for at least three years. Most single malts are matured longer. Barley, yeast and water are the only ingredients required in its production. The only additive allowed is natural caramel coloring.

Master Blender Richard Patterson, "The Nose" – insured on 8 million dollars – , as he is friendly known in the trade, is the brilliant production supervisor of the two most appreciated single malts in the international market, "The Dalmore" and "Jura".In our last encounter in Miami, Richard offered me the opportunity to taste some of these unique single malts. Let's elaborate:

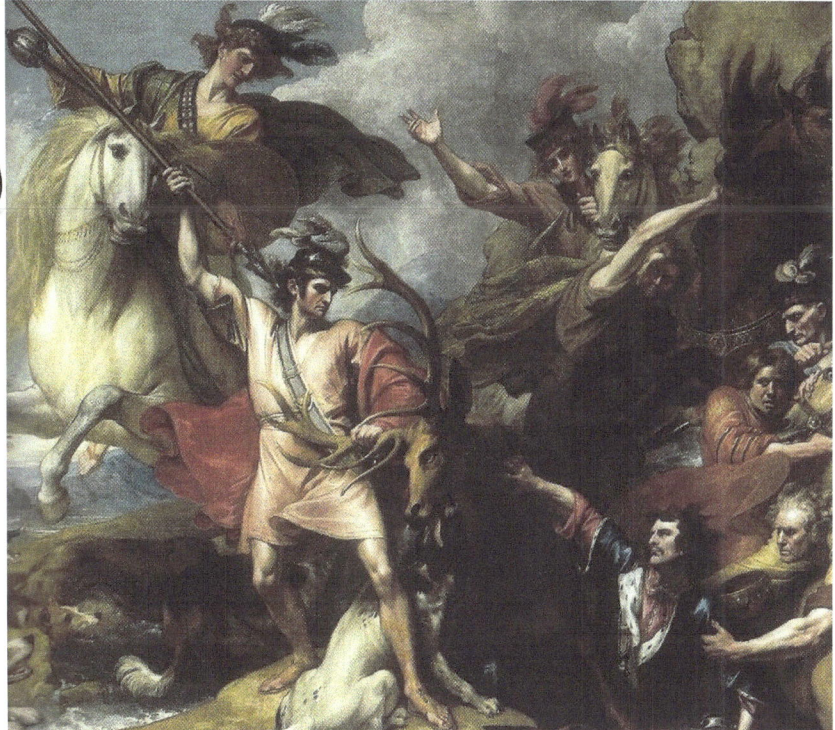

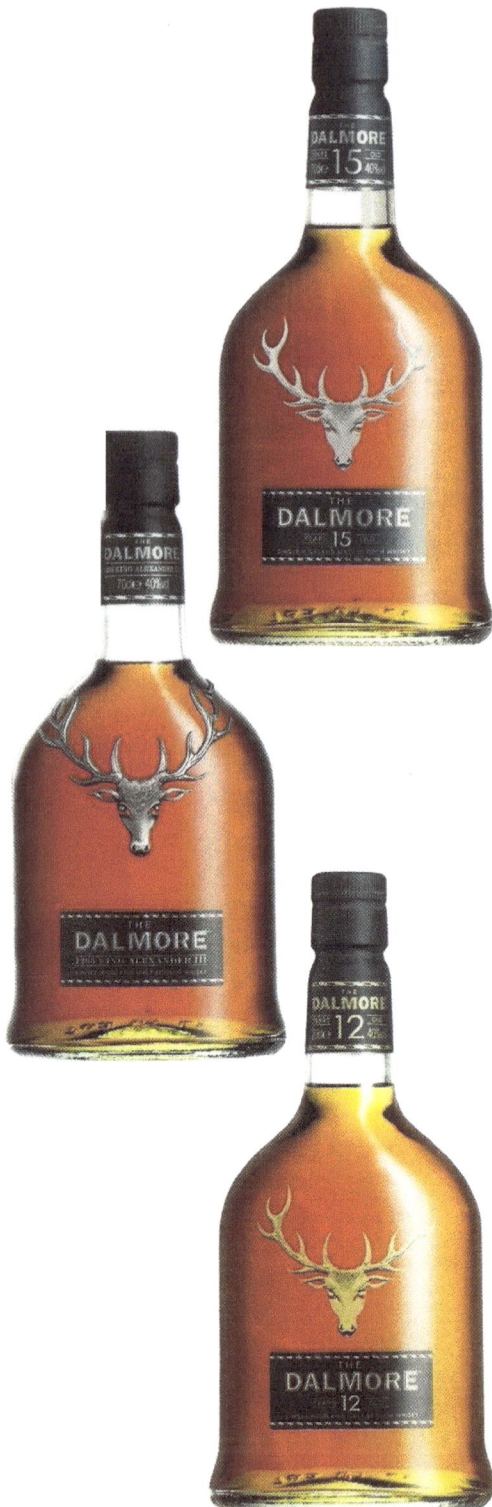

"**The Dalmore**". Legendary lineage of Scotland's culture: "The Dalmore" is a single highland malt whisky forged from its unique heritage and it owes its inception and development to a more dynamic and daring age. Sir Alexander Matheson was a partner in the dynastic Hong Kong commercial firm Jardine Matheson & Co, traders in everything from tea to opium and, of course, whisky. In 1839 Matheson purchased Ardross Farm, a Scotland mill sympathetically converted to a malt distillery. From 1886 the distillery was worked by tenants, the Mackenzie family, who were able to acquire the property launching The Dalmore brand. Centuries before, in 1263, an ancestor of the Clan Mackenzie, in a selfless act of courage, had saved King Alexander III from being gored by a stag in a hunting incident and the grateful King granted him the right to use the 12 points stag emblem in the MacKenzie coat of arms, decorating to the present day all their whisky bottles. These are the jewels of the collection:

THE DALMORE 1263 King Alexander III – This remarkable spirit has been filled to French Cabernet Sauvignon barriques, Madeira drums, sherry butts from Jerez, Sicilian Marsala barrels, Port pipes from the Douro and Bourbon barrels from Kentucky. The King Alexander III unites each of these to create an exceptional malt. Bouquet: tropical fruits, berries, vanilla.

THE 18 YEARS OLD – Matured initially in American white oak for 14 years before being transferred to
Matusalem Spanish sherry butts for 3 years, these unique whiskies were finally married for a further 12 moths in upstanding sherry butts. Bouquet: spice, chocolate, coffee.

THE 15 YEARS OLD – For this Dalmore, 15 years in bespoke Matusalem, Apostoles and Amoroso sherries from Jerez de La Frontera have all been elemental. The redolence of these vessels delivers the perfect balance between spirit, wood and maturity.

Bouquet: citrus, spices, orange.

THE GRAN RESERVA: This spirit offers a lively, youthful expression of single malt whisky derived from the combination of 60% sherry wood and 40% American white oak-aged malts ranging from 10 to 15 years of age. Firm and spirituous. Bouquet: citrus, dried fruits, chocolate, sherry, vanilla oak.

THE 12 YEARS OLD: Judicious selection and the precise balance of American white oak and Oloroso sherry wood deliver its most vibrant expression. Robust- yet elegant, with an aftertaste of brilliant complexity. Bouquet: spice, citrus, vanilla.

The Isle of "Jura". Magic and mystery in a bottle: There is no quick way of getting to the island of Jura.

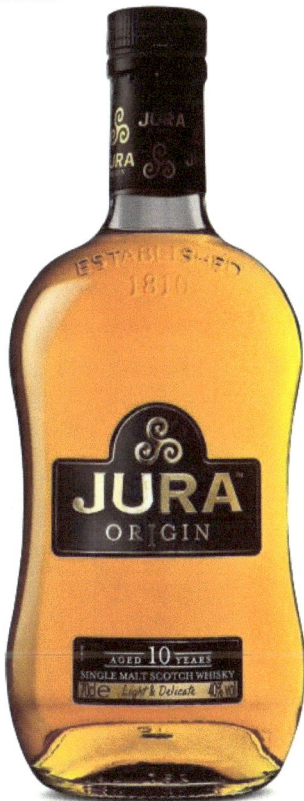

The fastest method from London involves two planes, a ferry, and the best part of a day. George Orwell, who came to Jura to write "1984 ", described it as "an extremely un-getable place". Things have not change a great deal since then, which is partly what makes this Hebridean island – producer of the award-winning JURA single malt – such a magical destination. Only 7 miles wide and 30 long, Jura is inhabited by 5,000 deer and about 200 people. Although private telephones were installed in the 1970's, replacing the island's three, don't expect to get a mobile phone signal, let along internet access. With one shop, one pub, a floating bank that comes once at week and its 180 year old distillery, it's "as good as life used to be", as the distillers like to say. For those who love the "great outdoors", Jura is an idyllic place, rich in history, myths and superstitions. Excavations show it welcomed some of the oldest settlements in Scotland over 8,000 years ago. It also became a Viking stronghold, while its ancient grave-yard boasts a number of Knights Templar grave stones.

But for true whisky enthusiasts there is an over-riding reason to come to Jura, and that is to visit its distillery. Established in 1810, JURA's single malts have won numerous awards. The island's exceptionally mild climate and gentle breezes, together with the local spring water, are significant factors contributing to JURA's smooth, warm and complex flavors. Presenting:

PROPHECY – The distinctive bottle features the "third eye" of a fabled seer who purportedly predicted the end of the Clan Campbell domination some 200 years before it occurred. With a burnished old gold color this whisky is a solera-style compendium of casks with varying levels of ageing. Rich, velvety mouth-feel, the spirit offers an intriguing mix of honey sweetness and dried fruits before turning drier with an intense pepper, nutmeg and cinnamon spice. Long peaty smoked final flavor.

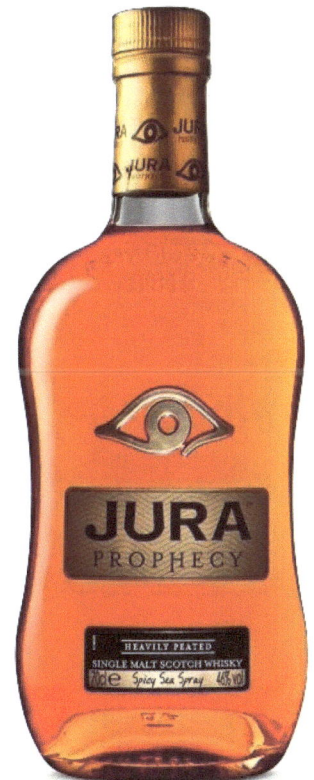

THE 16 YEAR OLD – These long years in American white oak will assist in raising the true depth of the spirit's quality. Aromas of silky marzipan honey with a hint of ginger spice and sweet chutney encompass this floral bouquet. Soft peaches and honey with tones of chunky orange peel and marzipan, together with hints of Napolean cognac, leave the palate rewarded and satisfied.

SUPERSTITION – Crafted from a selection of the finest aged Jura single malt whiskies (13 and 21 years old), "the bottled should be totally consumed the day is opened", says the legend. The Cross of Ankh, displayed on the bottle, will bring you health and good fortune if the elixir is served pressing firmly the palm of the hand to the Cross. Spice, honey, pine and peat aromas make a dramatic impact. Long persistent final.

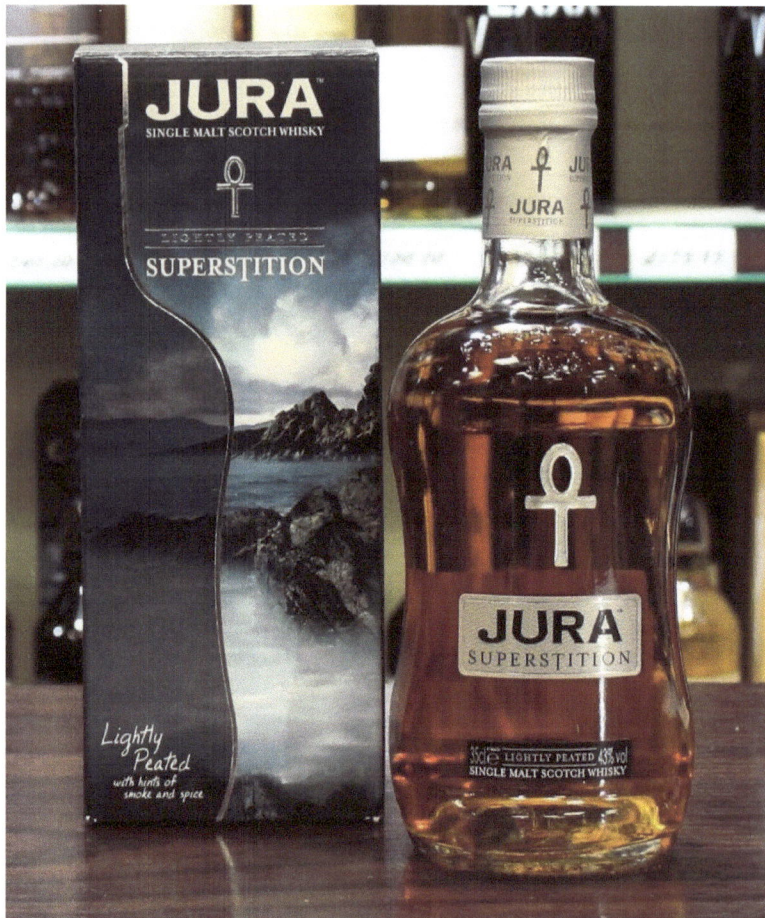

THE 10 YEAR OLD – The first distilled whisky in the island. Soft warm nuances of American oak, cinnamon and crushed pear and apple express their attractive qualities. Silky almond, pinewood and lemon grass complete this outstanding bouquet. Highlights of caramel, soft licorice and flashes of roasted coffee excite and tease your taste buds.

The best for the Holidays !

FRANCIS FORD COPPOLA, THE 'GODFATHER" OF WINE
Cinema and enology mastered by a brilliant mind

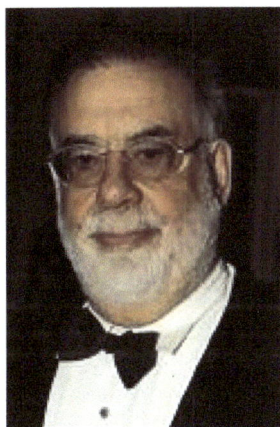

Son of Carmine Coppola, the remarkable composer and musician from Napoli, Francis was born in Detroit, but is in New York – particularly in Queens and Long Island – where he grew-up and lived most of his adolescence and early adulthood. During his infancy, Coppola became the family editor of all the household's 8 mm. movies. In 1955 received a P.H.D in Drama from Hofstra University in New York, followed by a degree in Cinematography and Film Production from the prestigious University of California at Los Angeles (U.C.L.A.). His dedication and talent allowed him to reach his professional debut at age 21 writing and directing his first feature film, "Dementia 13", in only 9 days ! , considered by Film Historians as the first on the "psychological terror" gender. It was in Ireland, during its filming, where he met Eleanor, the love of his life. They soon got married. The rest is a history of success, inspiration, awards and the winning of five Oscars from the Hollywood Film Academy. His classic corleonesque trilogy, "The Godfather" (1971), "II" (1974) and "III" (1990) has been universally recognized as the most acclaimed films of all times, superseding the moving epic "Gone with the Wind".

Coppola's deeply rooted Italian idiosyncrasy brought in him the delight of foods and wines of a typical Neapolitan family table. Agostino Coppola, Francis grandfather, was a winemaker and crafted his table wine in the basement of his Lexington Avenue apartment. In 1975, following his inspiration, joined his wife Eleanor on what became his other passion in life purchasing part of the Inglenook Vineyards, in the Rutherford district of Napa, California, with the intention of producing wines for domestic consumption. Eleanor, son Roman and daughter Sofia were the pillars of the vineyard, focusing their energy on earning and mastering the Organic Agriculture methods. "Movies and Winemaking have obvious similarities" – writes Coppola in Zoetrope, his literary magazine – "Both start with the primal matter. In the wine case are earth and grapes; in cinema, the story and the actors quality. The grapes can be affected by good or bad weather; the actors performance relies on many factors. The winemaker begins with the fermentation process and blending creativity, approving or discarding grape groups. The Director does the same, simply issuing a 'yes' or 'no' referring to cast, wardrobe, edition and sound mixing.

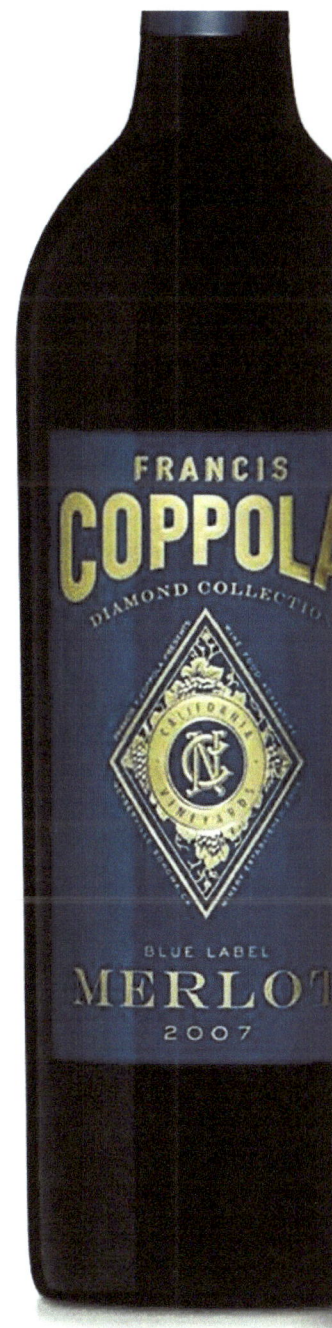

However, in both cases, you have to start with the best foundation, whether is the land or the script. Of course, on some instances, you just improvise and let Nature take its course. It's all entertainment".

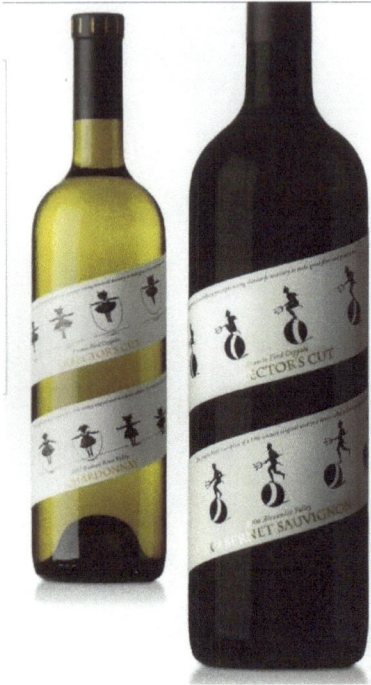

In the Inglenook vineyards, the first Cabernet Sauvignon plantings took place in 1882, nurtured by its founder Gustave Niebaum. Mother Nature allowed to preserve this vines as the source of great quality California wines. The Copolla family and there to date closer adviser, winemaker Corey Beck, launched their first ecological line under the name of "Niebum-Coppola Diamond Collection", honoring the old pioneer. In 2006, part of this property, 235 acres in fact, was converted exclusively for organic vine cultivation and renamed Rubicon Estate. That very same year, the illustrious Chateau Souverain Winery in Sonoma was purchased by the Coppolas, giving birth to their unique "Director's Cut" Selection. Soon after, honoring his daughter for the writing and directing Oscar winning film "Lost in Translation", Coppola launched the "Sofia Collection" presenting to the consumer a fresh sparkling Blanc de Blancs, a Rosé of grand style and an aromatic Riesling. All three sourced from the temperate vineyards of northern Monterey Peninsula, a region enveloped by cool marine conditions guaranteeing ripe and juicy berries with bright acidity.

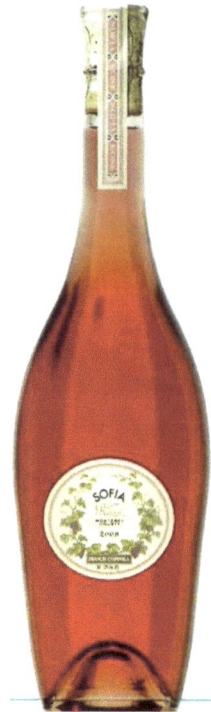

"The art of lodging" is something Coppola first intended in the 80s. The family has been building for the "enjoy life to the fullest" world's crowd, a stylish collection of three elite resorts in the coast of Belice, adjacent to Guatemala, inspired by the naturally beautiful surroundings of the Philippines, where his masterpiece Apocalypse Now was filmed. The Blancaneaux Lodge, Turtle Inn and La Lancha are a vivid example of a fervent eco-tourim. As a complement to all his creative "opuses", the family also celebrates the Italian traditions offering to the consumer the products of Coppola Brands, handling pasta and sauces creations, olive oil and balsamic vinegars among others.

Reviewing Francis Ford Coppola "other world":

THE GREATEST WINE IN HISTORY?
"Domaine Clarence Dillon" proudly presents CHATEAU HAUT-BRION

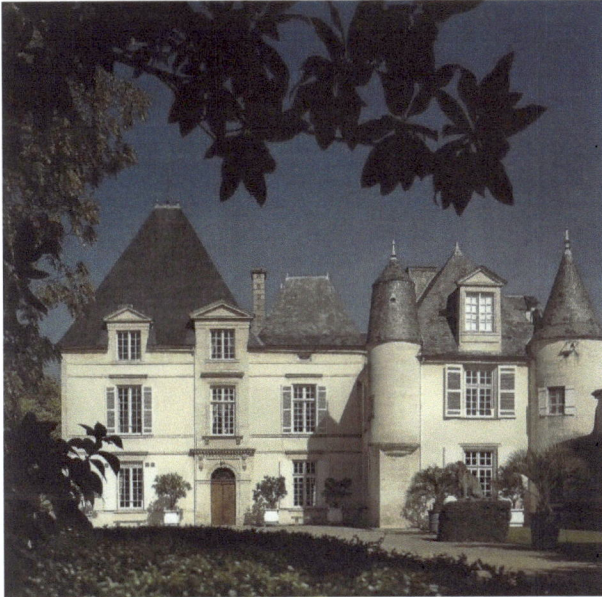

This illustrious estate is located in Pessac, region of Graves and just one mile from the city of Bordeaux. The estate devotes to wine 109 acres producing 12,000-15,000 cases annually and is planted with 55% Cabernet Sauvignon, 25% Merlot and 20% Cabernet Franc. The average age of vines is 35 years, been its wine rated as Grand Premier Cru Classé (Grand First-Growth). Is the only first-growth to be American owned and Bordeaux's first internationally acclaimed winemaking estate. Although grapes are thought to have been grown on the property since Roman times, the earliest document indicating cultivation of a parcel of land dates from 1423.

Chateau Haut-Brion dates back to 1525 when Jean de Pontac married Jeanne de Bellon who brought to him

in her dowry the land of Haut Brion. Illustrious owners have marked Haut Brion for more than four centuries: admirals, an archbishop, a Grand Marshal of France, a Governor of Guyenne, three mayors of Bordeaux, Charles-Maurice de Tayllerand, Minister of the French Government and, more recently, the Ambassador of the United States in Paris, Clarence Douglas Dillon, who was also Minister of Finance in the U.S. when J.F.Kennedy was President. As an interesting historical note, in 1877, Thomas Jefferson, then Minister to France, came to Bordeaux visiting Haut Brion and its amazing terroir. Enjoying immensely its experience, the wine became the first recorded first-growth to be imported to the United States when Jefferson purchased six cases during the travels and had them sent back to his estate in Virginia. Today, Prince Robert de Luxembourg, great-grand son of Mr. Dillon, has been presiding the Domaine since 2008.

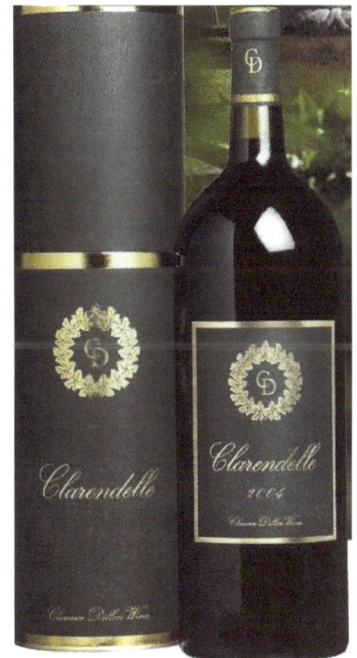

The selection of optimum rootstocks and clones has been a large task at Chateau Haut-Brion, pioneered by winemaker Jean-Bernard Delmas, which has greatly contribute to the quality of the plant material in the vineyard, ensuring healthy and balanced vines. Harvesting takes place by hand and each parcel is worked by the same team to increase their familiarity with the individual vines. The Grand Vin at Chateau Haut-Brion is fermented in stainless steel vats and aged in new oak barrels for 24 to 27 months. The winemaking, always managed by Mr. Delmas, is the result of a controlled but rather hot, short fermentation. The achievement is that of a wine with a complex bouquet of ripe fruit, tobacco and mineral earthy scents. Rich, ripe, medium to full-bodied and well structured. A wine that seems to balance perfectly power and elegance, richness and harmony An excellent complement to beef, lamb, veal and game.

Prince Robert de Luxembourg, in order to commemorate the 75th. Anniversary of the Domaine, ordered from a cabinetmaker of the English firm Linley Furniture Designers a true masterpiece in precious wood that will continue the tradition of the craftsmanship and prestige at Chateau Haut-Brion. Displayed in this artisanal console – only 15 were made – you find bottles of the finest vintages of its history:

1935 – 1945 (one of the last bottles) – 1959 – 1961 – 1975 – 1989 – 1990 – 2009.

Currently these are the wines produced by Domaine Clarence Dillon:
ROUGE Chateau Haut-Brion – Premiere Grand Cru Classé. "The King"
La Clarence de Haut-Brion – Second label red wine.
Chateau La Mission Haut-Brion – Cru Classé de Graves en Rouge.

La Chapelle de la Mission Haut-Brion – Second label red wine.
Chateau Qvintus Rouge 2011 & Le Dragon de Qvintus – First vintage of this two new reds.

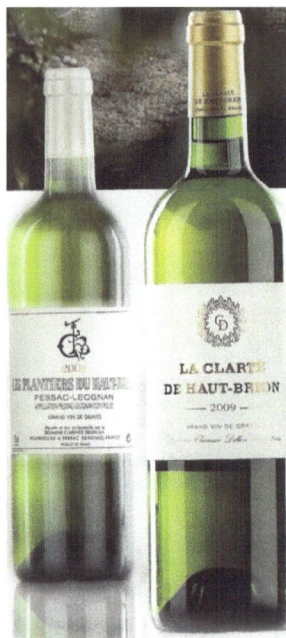

BLANC
Chateau Haut-Brion Blanc – The Traditional.
Chateau La Mission Haut-Brion Blanc – Second label to Chateau La Mission Haut-Brion.
La Clarté de Haut-Brion – Second label to Chateau Haut-Brion Blanc.
CLARET
Clarendelle – Launched in 2005 following the Claret style.

Santé pour tous!

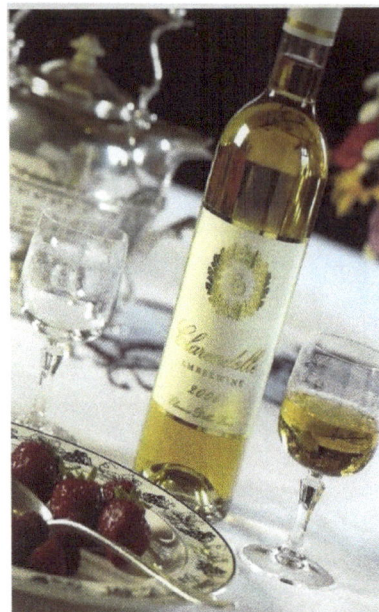

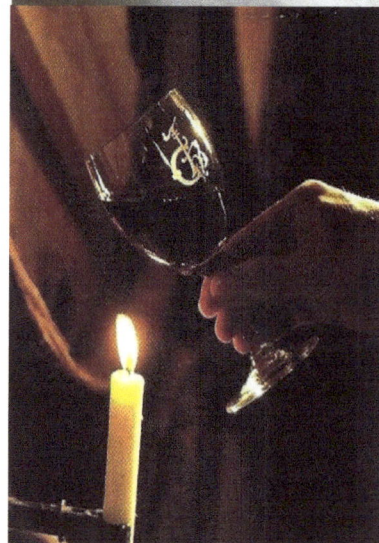

CUVÉES DE PRESTIGE
The deluxe wines of the Champagne Houses

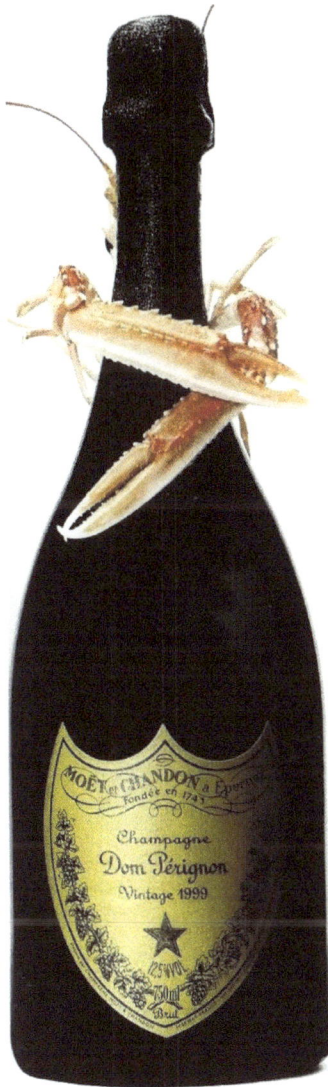

"Wine of Kings. King of Wines", the ultimate description of the nectar from Champagne. Is the invigorating and erotic bubbly, the legendary drink of the elite, the undisputed quality sparkling wine. From l'état c'est moi Louis XIV to the Czars of Russia, from Winston Churchill to the English royal family, Formula One winners to stock market flotations, the sparkling wine from the northernmost wine region of France is always present with anticipation, surrounding a spirit of refinement, voluptuousness, delicacy, exuberance and sensuality presiding in every sphere of life, from the salon to the boudoir. Unlike any other wine, it has establish its appellation as a brand name with which the greatest prestige – and the highest prices! – are inextricably linked.

Our purpose is not other but to present a small collection of the top Cuvées de Prestige, bottled only in years of outstanding characteristics offering the most brilliant vintages of recent market history. Champagne is compatible with all sorts of cuisine, pairing exemplary with moluscs, crustaceous, all types of fish, fowl, white meats, cheeses and, of course, with caviar, its eternal companion.

Dom Pérignon: In 1668, the young monk Pierre Pérignon, a man endowed with amazing intuition and foresight, took up his duties as cellar master at the Benedictine Hautvillers Abbey, in the western hills of the Marne river. For forty-seven years he worked on creating, perfecting and establishing the reputation of what later be known as the "Champagne" method. The House of Moet&Chandon, in Epernay, adopted his name, launching this Cuvée de Prestige in 1745.

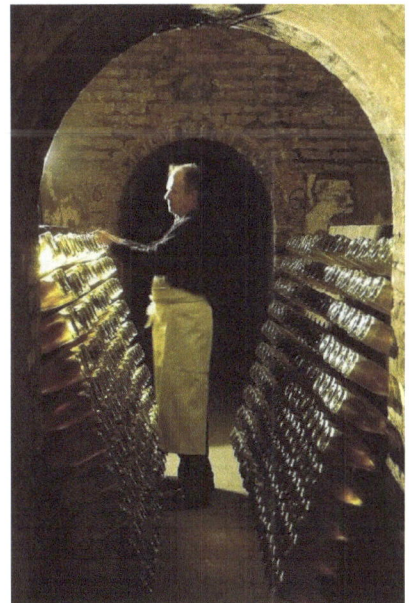

Dom Pérignon 1999: The latest vintage of extraordinary characteristics:
COLOR: Light golden with sunny radiance. Comes alive in a light, playful spiral. AROMA: Touches of coconut, cinnamon, cocoa and tobacco. BOUQUET: In the mouth, the wine reaches a state of complex fullness: earthy, smoky and pearly, underscored by the vibrant warmth of peppery spice. Intensity develops with a fruity, exotic maturity with a long finish.

Dom Pérignon Rosé 1996 – With this magnificent champagne the very idea of luxury and sensuality is taken to its peak. COLOR: Shades of amber, orange, copper and gold. The wonderful paradox is that this rosé is never pink. AROMA: The essence of malt rapidly leads into that of well-ripened fruit, nectarine and strawberries, complemented by smoky, peaty accents. BOUQUET: Brings to the palate an affirmation of boldness and authority with a slight vanilla-spicy note underscored in its firm and sharp finish.

Louis Roederer Cristal: The company is founded in Reims in 1776. A hundred years later Alexander II, Czar of Russia, names Louis Roederer his personal cuvée ordering a special bottle for him. That is haw "Cristal" was born in the Russian Court. Right after Louis Roederer inherits the business from his uncle. He gives the firm his own name and, under his leadership, it develops rapidly. Today is regarded as the ultimate premium champagne.

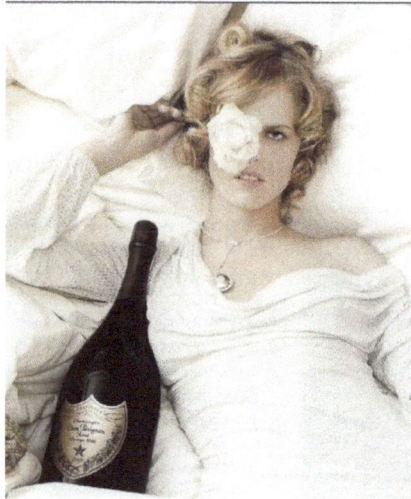

Cristal Vintage 2000: You can assert its finesse, balance and aromatic complexity. Ripe, precise and persistent but also light, refined and masterfully subtle. COLOR: Sustained golden yellow tones with luminous green highlights and ultra-fine, lively bubbles. AROMA: Opens with dominant aromas of fresh almonds and sweet-smelling flowers revealing nuances of lush peaches, white chocolate, caramel and lightly toasted hazelnuts.

BOUQUET: An almost caressing mouth feel supported by a refreshing crispness, giving you an impression of delicacy rather than strength. The finish is long with light caramel notes.

Champagne Krug: It was founded in 1843 by Johann-Joseph Krug in order to concentrate on the high end of the Champagne market. The traditions of Krug have been handed down from generation to generation, and today Olivier and Caroline Krug are taking over for their fathers Henri and Rémi Krug. Production varies from year to year, but in general is around 500,000 bottles of all types for the entire world, a miniscule production, but the very finest, bar none. The Krugists International Private Club is the most exclusive brotherhood in the world for Champagne lovers.

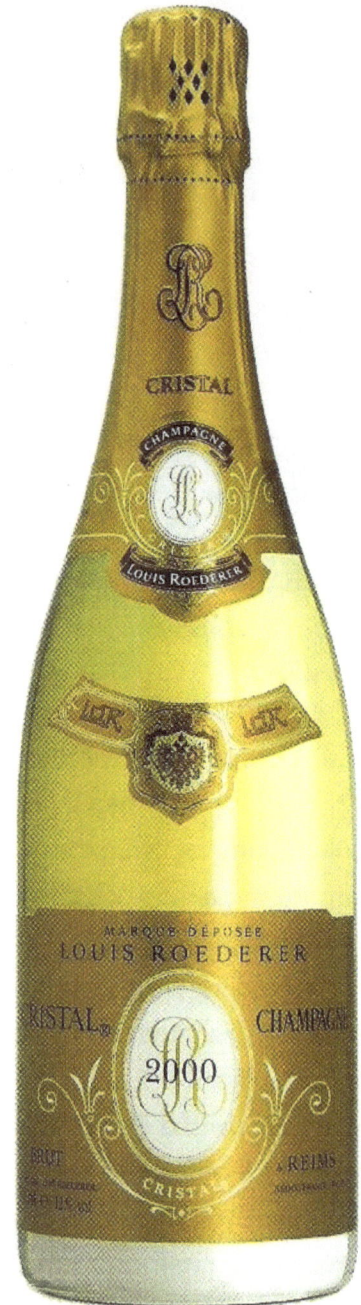

Krug Grand Cuvée 1996: The House of Krug presents this vintage year, widely considered the best of the twenty century in Champagne A highly changeable summer, alternating periods of scorching heat with spells of heavy rain, was followed, as harvest approached, by dry, sunny days and unusually chilling nights, which nurtured wines of contrast and character. The notably selection of grapes and the art of blending by Krug artisans also contributed to the excellence of this wine. We also want to mention the outstanding Krug 1990, almost impossible to find today. COLOR: Rich, radiant gold. AROMA: Full, ripe flavors, exploding into freshness. BOUQUET: A rainbow of essences. Fresh pear, candied lemon, ripe fruit, honey, gingerbread, mocha.

Krug 1990. Almost impossible to find in the market

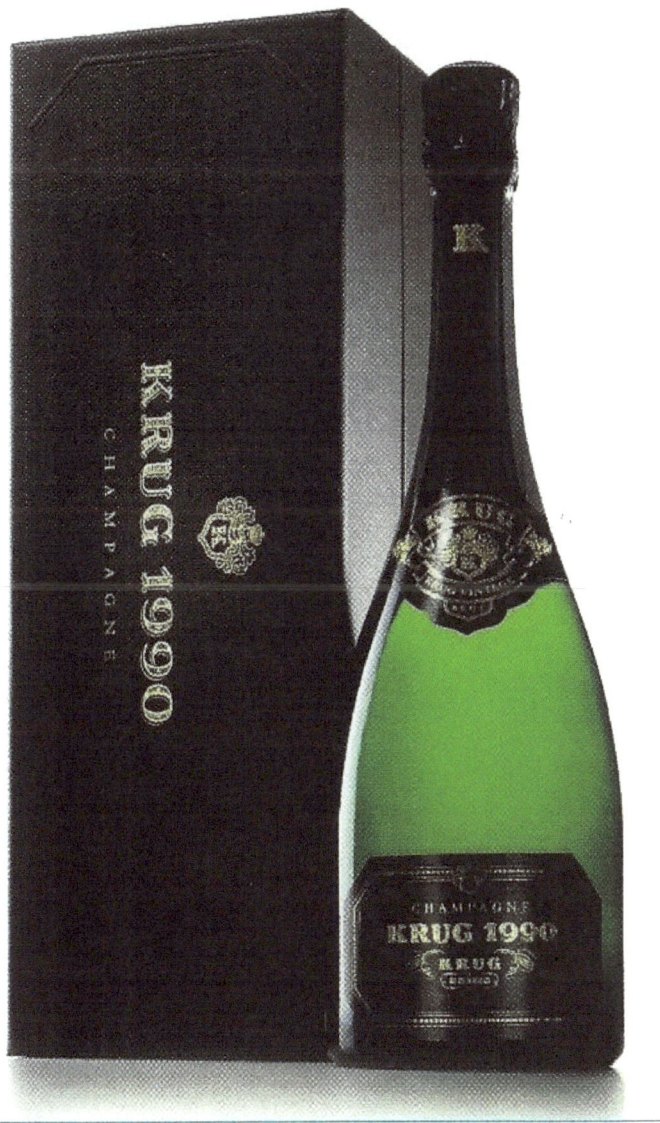

La Grande Dame: The Jewel of Clicquot. Legendary for its quality, the wine is made exclusively from eight Grands Crus vineyards purchased by Madamme Clicquot herself in Reims and favored for over two centuries by the House of Veuve Clicquot, whose passion, genius and tenacity made her wines world famous and gave her the nickname, "La Grande Dame de la Champagne".

Veuve Clicquot La Grande Dame 1996 : An incomparable finesse created from the blend of the eight historic Grands Crus, aged for extended time in the ancient chalk cellars. Extreme fine effervescence with a distinctive fragrance of blending harmoniously both aromas and nobility. A silky mouth perfectly balanced with structure and dynamism of 65% Pinot Noir and 35% Chardonnay. COLOR: Intensely golden. AROMA: Notes of lemon, honey and coffee. BOUQUET: Subtle aspects of biscuit and whole-grain bread. Wonderful finesse and harmony underscore its innate power and vinosity. An extremely long and uniquely aromatic finish.

Dom Ruinart: Back in 1729, when Nicolas Ruinart laid the foundations of the very first Champagne House, he was in fact realizing the ambition of his uncle Dom Thierry Ruinart, a Benedictine monk considered in the History of Wine as one of the most brilliant promotional minds in the Worl of Champagne.

A visionary and enlightened pioneering spirit, he intuitively foresaw the fame and commercial success this wine would enjoy in the future. Invited to Versailles, he noted the Court's enthusiasm for Champagne and shared his insight with his nephew Nicolas well known as an ambitious entrepreneur who finally launched the Ruinart family into the great adventure of champagne trading.

The House is now represented all over the world and its champagne is considered a masterpiece paying tribute to the vision of its inspired founder.

Dom Ruinart 1996: With the typical characteristics of the 1996 harvest, this vintage is indeed worthy of the esteemed Dom Ruinart lineage. Ready for drinking now, this champagne will never fail to enchant.

You, however, it can also be laid down in a good wine cellar for a tasting in a few years' time. Through Time, this prestige vintage will continue to astound you. COLOR: Golden yellow with delicate bronze highlights with a fine long lasting effervescence. AROMA: Notes of white flowers, citrus and also tropical fruits such as lychee. BOUQUET: Subtle and silky in the palate revealing notes of grapefruit and passion fruit with an excellent lingering crisp finish.

Try them all!

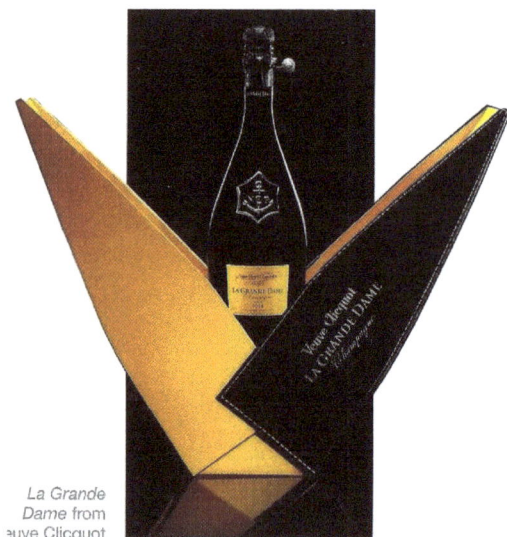

La Grande Dame from ?uve Clicquot

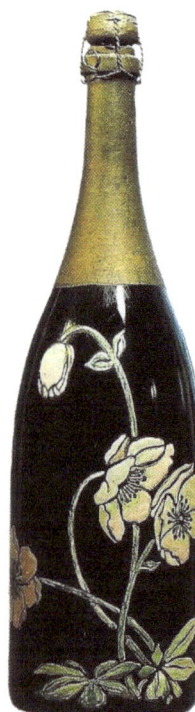

Original design of the Fleur de Champagne bottle by Emile Gallé

THE WINES FROM TORO

The most sough-after of Spain

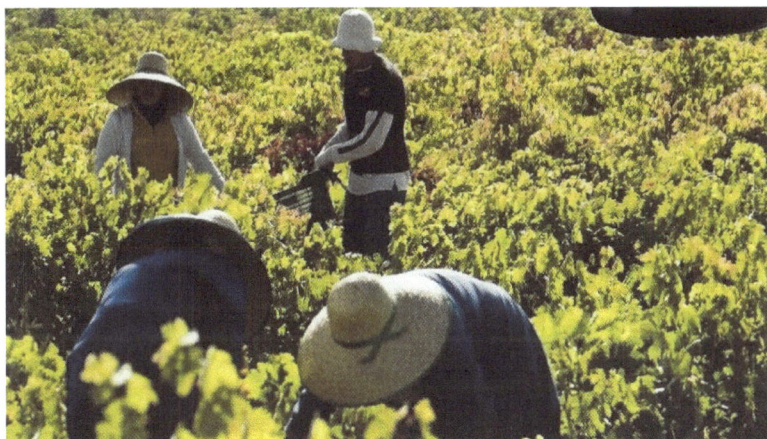

The production area for the wines of Toro lies at the western extremity of the Castilla y Leon region, in Noth-Western Spain. This is a place of long-standing wine-making traditions, as the vineyards go back to Ancient Roman times. During the Middle Ages, these wines were enjoyed all over the Spain, due to the intense trading, encouraged by a royal privilege. Taken on board of Spanish fleets, wines from Toro were also part of the New World adventure. Later, at the end of the 19th century, the region's wines were exported to other European countries hard hit by Phylloxera crisis, given that the Toro vines are naturally immune to the plague.

The use of the geographical designation "Toro" was officially recognized in 1933. The "Denominación de Origen" was born in 1987 and strict regulations were established for its management. Today, this viticultural region covers an area of 62,000 hectares in the South-East of the province of Zamora.

Rising in the Ribera del Duero region, the River Duero crosses the Toro area, flowing westwards and becoming the Douro after crossing the border with Portugal, where it shapes the vineyards that also produce the Port wines.

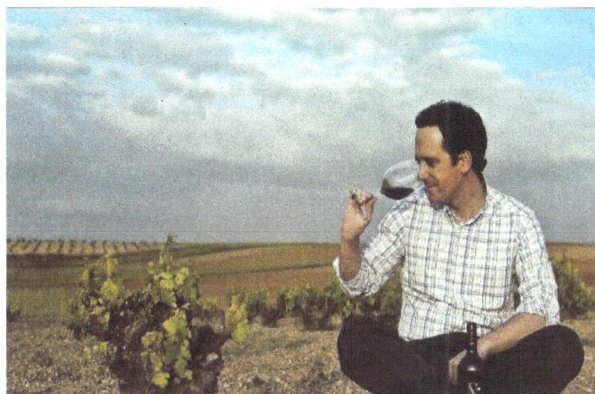

Most Toro wines are made from a single grape variety called "Tinta de Toro", part of the Tempranillo family. The Duero River and its tributaries have formed the landscape, sculpting the hills that lie at between 650 and 850 meters above sea-level. The vineyards are sited on the plateau or the slopes of this high ground and the climate is continental with an oceanic influence. Ownership is shared amongst 1,200 different growers involved in grape cultivation and wine production, however I am going to present two top wineries symbolizing a rare combination of classicism and innovation.

Let's elaborate:

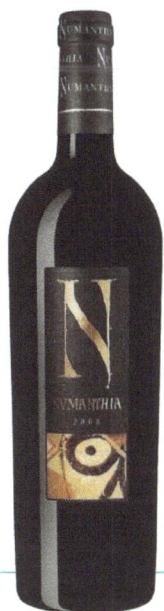

BODEGA NUMANTHIA: The name associates the ancient celticiberian town of

79

Numancia, known in Old History for their resistance to the Roman invaders. After 20 years of hostilities, in the year 133 BC, the Roman Empire gave Scipio Aemilianus Africanus the task of destroying Numancia. After 13 months of siege, the Numanthians decided to burn the city and die free rather than live and be slaves. Its ruins have been preserved as a symbol of heroism. The estate was founded in 1998 by the Eguren Family, from the Rioja region. From the start their aim of Marcos and Miguel Eguren was to produce the best wine from Toro, compatible with all types of dishes and styles of cuisine.

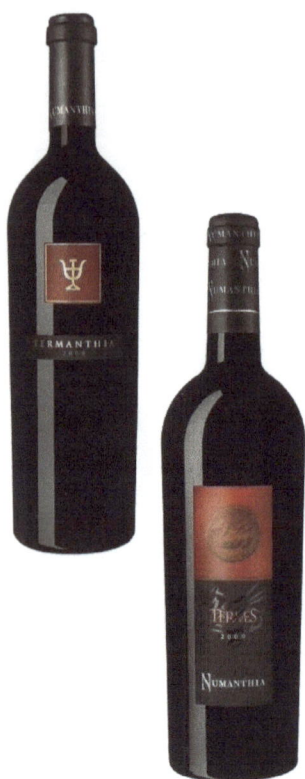

Termes: The Termes grapes are selected for their intense, vibrant and lively fruit expression. A wine, perfect adaptation of the Tinta de Toro vines, revealing classy and intense aromas, rich and complex flavors with abundant fruity notes integrated with hints of cedar and toasty characters. Numanthia: This wine's style relies on a selection of exceptional ungrafted old vineyards, with more than 50 years. These low yielding vines offer, year after year, extreme grapes concentration, fruit intensity and structure. Solidly built, with tannins that are both sharp and well integrated, Numanthia expresses power, precision and persistence. The wine of "ancient heroes".

Termanthia: The meticulous elaboration of this wine is the ultimate expression of the 120 year old best vineyard plots of the region.

To create wine with this unique grapes is a matter of hand-crafting excellence.
The sublime fruit concentration unveils a magnificent aromatic complexity that reveals as much intensity as precision and elegance.

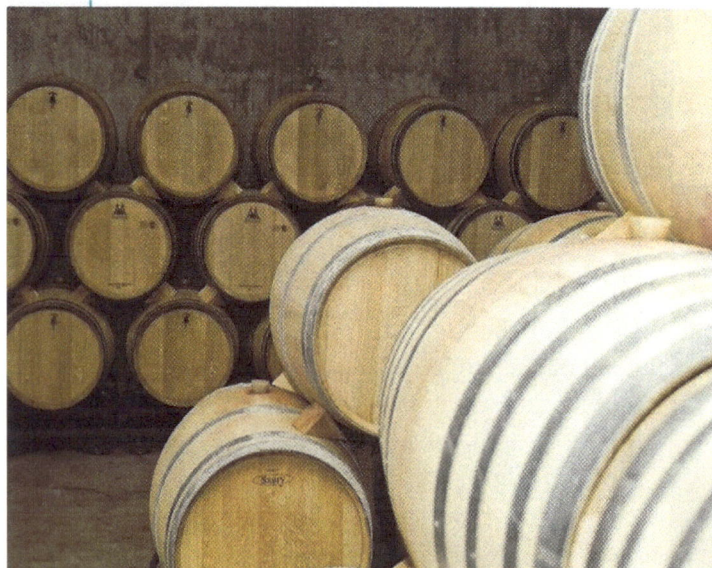

THE BEAUTY OF WINE DECANTING

A sign of respect for old wines and of confidence in young wines

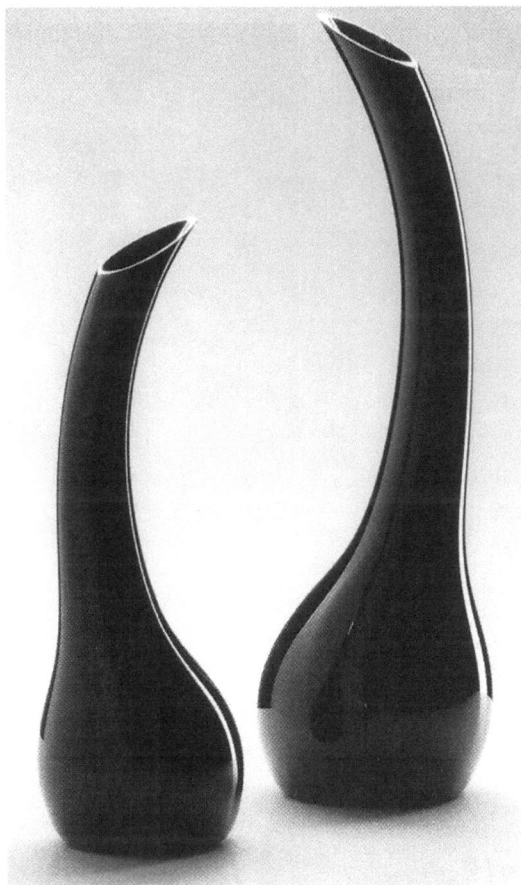

Decanting has become de rigueur in fine restaurants and many aficionados and wine lovers have added decanters to their collection of wine accoutrements at home. Is not only highly decorative for the table but a real necessity to obtain the highest clarity, perfect bouquet and a maximum texture enhancement of wine. Christian Mouiex, owner of the legendary Chateau Petrus says, "Decanting old wines, just a few moments before they are served, helps ensure that the wine's brilliance is not obscured by any sediments that may have developed over time. Decanting young wines, several hours before serving them, gives the wine a chance to bloom and obtain a stage of development that normally requires years of aging". An elegant decanter adds immensely to the beauty of the dinner table and heightens the expectation that the wine will be delicious.

No one within the wine world has better attained this target that Maximilian Josef Riedel, CEO of RIEDEL CRYSTAL AMERICA and the 11th generation carrier of a traditional excellence in design and artisanal production of the finest, most appreciated, wine and spirits lead crystal ware marvels. Together with his father Georg, the House of Riedel developed – besides the finest classic glassware for the dinner table, a decanters collection, complex in design and free hand blown (as opposed to being blown into a mold) in their Austrian factory. Only the most experienced glass artist can create these unorthodox pieces and, like all great art, each decanter is truly one of a kind named individually by inspiration. Let us run through the most distinguish examples:

"AMADEO": Introduced in 2006 to commemorate Riedel's 250th anniversary. Shaped like a lyre, this decanter has become an instant classic. A limited edition in black crystal was later added. "O" THMBS UP decanter, conceived exclusively by Maximilian. The ergonomic design with its deep punt, nestles comfortably in your hand and its perfect balance makes pouring effortless. He also designed the "CORNETTO" ("bugle" in Italian). His inspiration for this vessel came while watching the swans at the Bellagio Hotel in Vegas, making him think that a very long-necked decanter would make it easier for wait staff when pouring wine at the table. The success of **Cornetto** gave birth to the **"Bird Series"** presented in three decanters: **"PALOMA"**, **"FLAMINGO"** and **"SWAN"**. Maximilian and Georg were inspired to create these shapes on a birthday trip to Venice, while observing the poetry of movement in the flight of a flock of birds over the Piazza San Marcos, across the summer skies. The curvilinear **Paloma** blurs the line between art and design, elevating wine presentation to new heights.

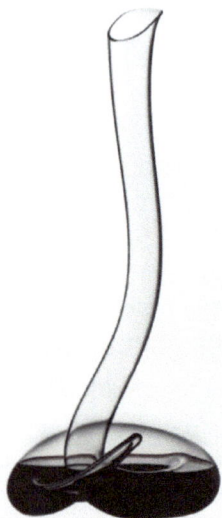

The **Flamingo** and the **Swan**, standing 23-5/8 inches tall, expose their natural grace and elegance making them a stunning *object d'art*. **"The Black Collection"**, recently developed, is clearly Riedel's most romantic line of decanters to date, baptized **SMILE, TOUCH** and **BLISS**. From a company where beauty and utility go hand-in-hand, these lustrous decanters are not only inspiring works of art, but practical pieces for everyday use that engage the senses with their dramatic design. With its soft curves, **Smile**'s inverted heart-shaped base makes it effortless to hold in the palm of the hand and easy to poor. Starting from the narrow opening at the top, its signature tuxedo line descends dramatically to the bottom. Seemingly defying gravity, **Touch** rests confidently on a bulb-shaped base and features a ridge adorned with a chic ribbon of black crystal guaranteeing a comfortable grip in the hand. A labor of love, **Bliss** displays a rotund foundation with an off-center heart stamped from each side, thus compressing the crystal into a thin pane of solid glass. Like the rest of the collection, Bliss is dressed up with a black tuxedo stripe that extends gracefully from top to bottom. With **"FACE TO FACE",** you will be able to enhance your wine profile combining function and fancy in the same product. This graceful, soaring decanter features two concave profiles facing one another in the interior of the vessel. By swirling vigorously the wine until a foam cap develops, it achieves the maximum effect of oxygen on young tannins.

The result is more satisfying, intense fruitiness on the mid-palate and a more rounded texture. And now is the moment to introduce **"EVE"**, a decidedly different decanter. The sensuous, serpentine curves of Riedel's newest mouth blown lead crystal decanter are not only seductive, but also functional. This design *tour de force*, double decants your wine as it flows through the coiled shape. Serving wine becomes a performance as the decanter's requires a slow 360 degree rotation to "charge" it and allow the wine to pour. **Eve** is a decanter that also speaks – it emits a sound akin to the gurgle of the King Cobra as the wine makes its trip through the curvaceous swirl of glass. Its long and graceful neck means that you can easily pour for a guest across the table without moving from your spot.

The **Eve** decanter, designed by Maximilian Riedel in 2008, is a tribute to the family's matriarch, Eva Riedel.
Enjoy your wines using the necessary art of decanting!

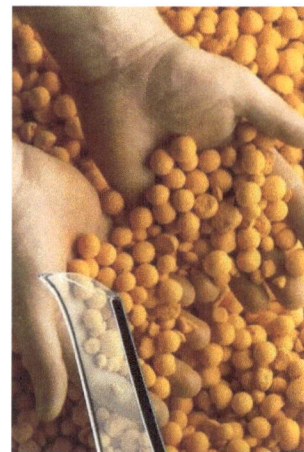

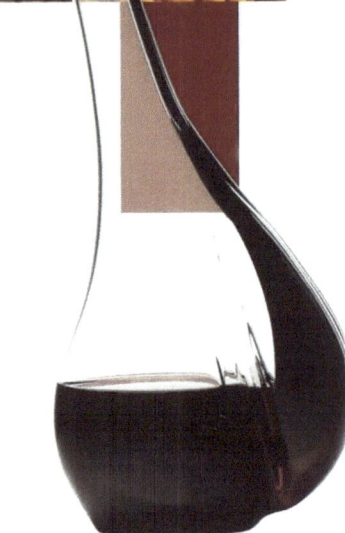

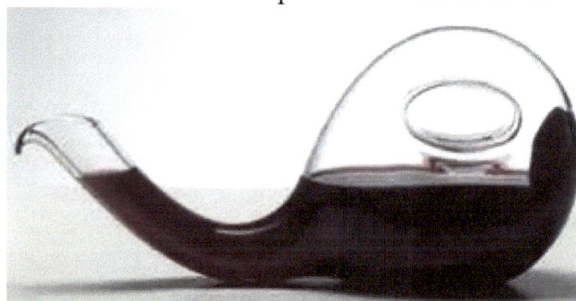

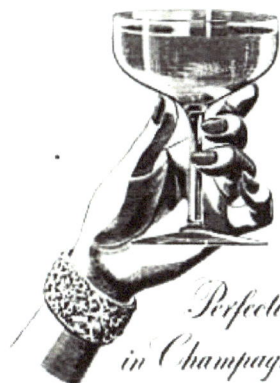

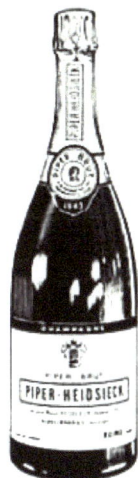

THE FAVORITE CHAMPAGNE OF QUEEN MARIE- ANTOINETTE
The "unconventional chic" PIPER HEIDSIECK

Once upon a time since 1785, Florens-Louis Heidsieck was the son of a Lutheran minister from Westphalia, who worked in Reims, France, as a cloth merchant. While living in Reims, he developed a passion for winemaking and began making his own champagne. Although he was neither a viticulturist nor a native of Reims – the universal capital of champagne making he displayed talent and worked at his profession founding his own Champagne House. Rigorous quality standards were developed by the House making sure that only the best grapes were used in its highly recognized champagnes. Heidsieck proudly dedicated his best Cuvée to Queen Marie-Antoinette and was granted the honor of personally presenting her with a bottle only a few months after founding his House. The Queen, – patron of the Arts and Fashion – impressed by the wine's excellence, adopted it immediately as the Champagne of the French Royal Court.

Intense, vibrant and elegant, it quickly enticed the neighboring European Courts. The whirlwind of the age of enlightenment sees the birth of Piper-Heidsieck, as a result of the encounter between Florens-Louis and the oenologist Henry-Guillaume Piper. The uniqueness of their philosophy "create very seriously wines that smile" will be at the core of the House spirit: a perfect balance between excellence and originality. In 1828 Henry-Guillaume Piper assume the control of the House, travels the world and becomes the official purveyor to 14 Royal and Imperial Courts, including those of Siam and China. Everybody asks for Piper-Heidsieck! In 1885, Karl Fabergé – leading proponent of the Art Déco movement and purveyor to the Imperial Court of Alexander III – opens up the doors of Russia for Piper-Heidsieck. by creating a bottle whose diamonds and gold were an homage to its sparkle. When in 1960, Marilyn Monroe declares that "she goes to bed with only a drop of perfume and wakes up with a flute of Piper-Heidsieck", she lends her natural glamour to Piper-Heidsieck's international conquest. In 1968 the House introduces the most expensive bottle of champagne in the world with a reedition of the wine created for Marie-Antoinette, using the same 12 crus utilized by Florens-Louise Heidsieck 1n 1785. Since it foundation, Piper-Heidsieck has never ceased to attract the most creative spirits, those who have shape their times and left an eternal trace. A unique, chic and irreverent positioning in Champagne.

Presenting the 2011 Piper-Heidsieck achievers of 1 GRAND GOLD Medal, 9 GOLD Medals, 8 SILVER Medals, 1 #1 CHAMPAGNE OF THE YEAR, 1 SPARKLING WINE OF THE YEAR and 1 FRENCH WINE OF THE YEAR :

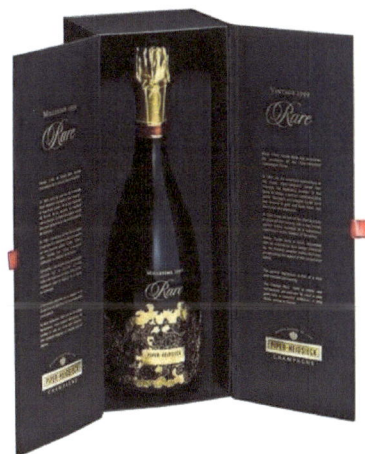

P–H BRUT N/V: On the eye – Sparkling clarity. Pale gold color. Bouquet – Bright and fresh first impressions. Reminiscent of spring blossoms leading to more fruity notes such as summer apple and pear then citrus with hints of warm toastiness. Palate – Lively and fresh. Citrus notes take on a certain maturity. Passion with gentleness, lightness with spontaneity. Food Pairings – This is the perfect social drink. Great with appetizers and cheeses. For the meal with chicken, pork or veal . Informal fish and seafood dinners and "nouvelle cuisine" surprises.

P-H ROSE SAUVAGE: On the eye – An intense, bright, deep pink color. Bouquet – Vivacity and passion fresh hints. Bouquet – Strong aromas of red fruits with cherries dominating. This leads to notes of citrus fruits, mandarin and blood orange. A final touch of cinnamon. Palate – A spirited, lively and full wine. Slight acidity lingering with hints of strawberry, plum, blood orange and an enthusiastic welcome sensation of warmth. Food Pairings – Cold and hot appetizers. Main courses of Rack of Lamb and Duck "a l'orange". Sweets: Raspberry/pistaccio macaroons. Peach/apricot on a sponge cake with fromage blanc cream.

P-H BRUT Vintage 2004: On the eye – A sunny yellow color showing a delicate bubble reinforcing the sparkle. Bouquet – A soft first impression of cereal, fresh almonds and hazelnuts leading to notes of apricot, rhubarb, ripe citrus and floral notes (roses, violets). Naturally elegant. A perfect balance of power and finesse. Palate – The firm and melting texture suggests a cocktail of dried exotic fruits, the coconut slightly enhanced by a touch of cedar wood. A subtle balanced wine that suggests eternal youth. The statue of a Greek athlete. Food Pairings – Cold appetizer of tomato and cucumber tartare with a sweet & sour sauce of yellow pepper. Hot appetizer of dried prunes wrapped in bacon. Cooked shrimp and pineapple brochette. Main course of grilled shrimp with fruit chutney and passion fruit sauce. Sweets, toffee/chocolate/vanilla macaroon.

P-H SUBLIME: On the eye – A warm copper shade with a joyous string of bubbles. Bouquet – At first a flowery touch of violet. Generous notes of dried fruit, caramelized pear, licorice, cinnamon and vanilla will follow. Palate – A freshness that gives place to an impression of a soft, round an mellow cuvee. There are notes of caramelized flambéed pineapple and a wide array of pastries. A finish of mild spices, vanilla and cinnamon offering a subtle balance between freshness and warmth. Food Pairings & Sweets – Follow similar suggestions for the P-H Brut Vintage 2004.

P-H RARE Vintage 2002: On the eye – Pale gold color with reflections of green. A subtle effervescence, yet vivacious. Bouquet – The first aroma is vegetal, complex, subtle, delicate and relatively discreet. Notes of vetiver and exotic wood, followed by pepper, ginger and cumin. Evocations of roasted coffee beans. The aromas reveal themselves one by one with a highly distinctive oriental finale, reminiscent of meant tea and incense. Palate – A radiant wine, refined and elegant. A light, tonic wine, showing richness and density. Various spices, both fresh and fiery reminiscent of peppers and ginger. The finale is long and delicate: A veil blowing in the fresh desert breeze. Fantastic surrounding a "Lawrence of Arabia" atmosphere party.

Always capable of re-inventing with style, Piper Heidsieck carries the signature of a Grande Maison de Champagne.

"MASI AGRICOLA" FROM THE ITALIAN "VENETO"
Indigenous grapes, spectacular wines and singular methods

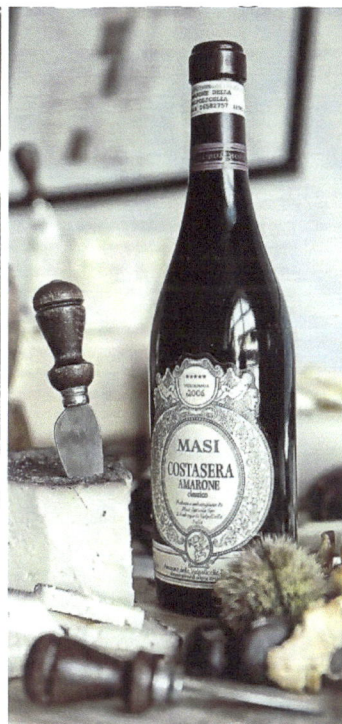

The name MASI comes from "Vaio dei Masi", a valley purchased by the Boscaini family in the late 18th Century. Rooted in the Veneto's history and tradition, "Masi Agricola" also manages the most historic estate in Valpolicella, wich once belonged to descendants of the legendary 14th Century poet Dante, from the noble Serego Alighieri family. "Masi Agricola"has also developed projects in Tuscany and Argentina. Viticulture is an integral part of the thousand-year-old inheritance of the Veneto region. Masi's viticultural expertise is a continuation of experience passed down by tradition and knowledge acquired from modern research. Of primary importance are the selection of specific vineyard sites, use of indigenous grape varieties and respect for historic winemaking techniques from Veneto.

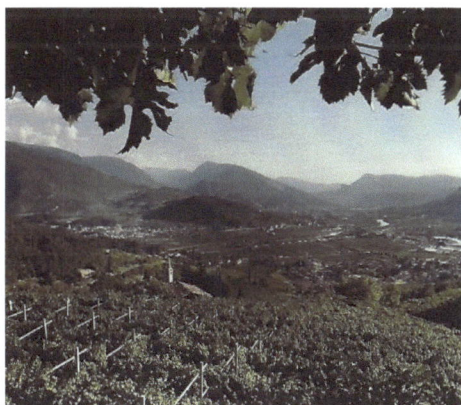

Appassximento is the traditional method used in the Veneto for concentrate aromas and flavors in wine. Before vinification, grapes are laid out on bamboo racks in drying lofts over the winter, an ancient technique used for centuries in the region. Passed down through generations of the Boiscani family, this craft has been modified in an innovative way by the Masi Technical Group and is used today to make fresh and lively wines from semi-dried grapes, notably Amarone the mother-grape of the most illustrious Italian wine. This method guarantees the authenticity and quality of Masi wines.

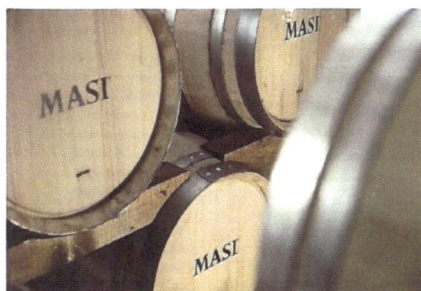

These are the three brilliant wines recognized all around the world:

Masianco Pinot Grigio e Verduzzo delle Venezie 2012 (75% Pinot Grigio, 25% Verduzzo):

Masi' most up-to-date Italian White is also the estate's white "Supervenetian", a wine of great personality. The wine blends the elgant, fruity and rich aromas of this grape with the structure, poise and body of the native Verduzzo grape , picked slightly over-ripe and mature.

Shows attractive, tropical fruit aromas. Fresh and charming palate flavors gain weight and become full on the mid-palate, where fruitiness blends with traces of honey and boiled sweets.

A dry finish has a citrus twist. Recommendations; An ideal aperitif, this wine is perfect with hors d'oeuvres, fish and white meats. This medium-bodied white has great personality, well suited for modern and oriental cuisine. Alcohol: 13.37%.

Campofiorin Rosso del Veronese 2010 (70% Corvina, 25% Rondinela, 5% Molinara): This wine is the original "Supervenetian" made with Masi's double fermentation technique.

A specialty wine, this red is made from local Veronese grapes vinified and then re-fermented with a small percentage of semi-dried grapes of the same varieties followed by malolactic.

Fruity cherry and plum aromas, with vanilla, cinnamon and spice notes. Shows sublime, soft tannins on the palate, with fresh acidity. Finish is long and persistent, with ripe fruit flavors and a touch of sweet spiciness. Recommendations: This versatile wine is perfect with various foods, including pastas with reach meats or mushrooms based sauces, grilled or roasted red meats, game and mature cheeses. Alcohol; 13.10%.

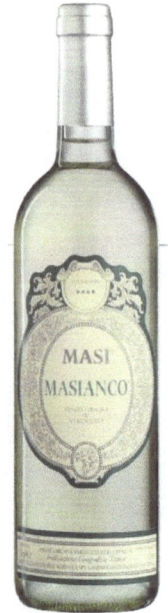

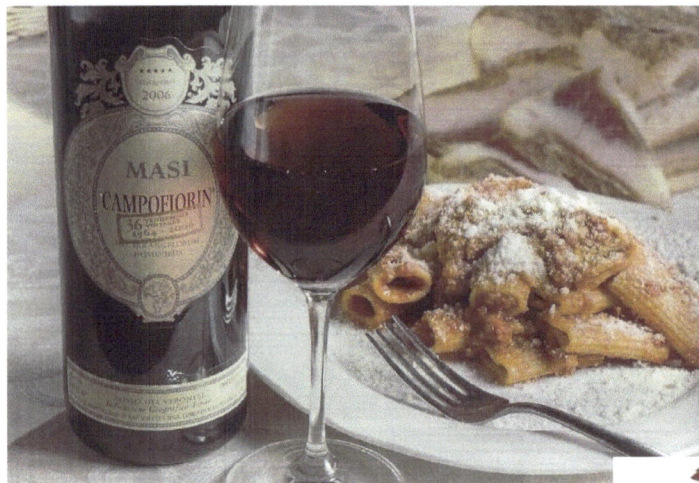

Costasera Amarone della Valpolicella Classico 2009 (70% Corvina, 25% Rondinella, 5% Moilnara): With sunset-facing slopes, Costasera is the best terroir for producing high quality Amarone in Valpolicella Classico. Wth a longer day, vines facing Lake Garda get reflected and direct sunlight, with soft breases. After gentle pressing, partially stemmed grapes undergo fermentation in large Slavonian oak barrels or stainless steel vats at low temperature.

Powerful, complex aromas of dried plums, with "balsamic" (anise, fennel, mint) traces. This wine is quite dry, soft and with bright acidity, with baked cherries, chocolate and cinnamon flavors and structured, noble tannins. Recommendations: Great with grilled or roasted red meats, game and hard cheeses. Considered "a wine for meditation", also to be sipped on its own or as a perfect after-dinner wine. Alcohol: 14.85%

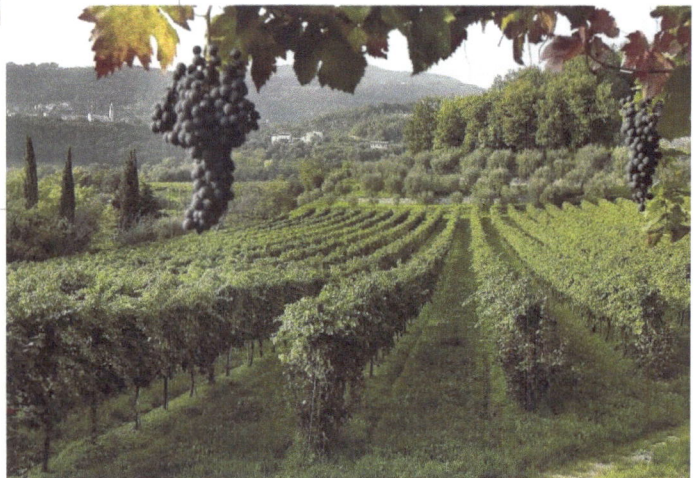

A true Italian Gift for the palate !

ELEGANCE AND CHARACTER FROM CALIFORNIA
"LAETITIA" and "NADIA" champion wines of class and diversity

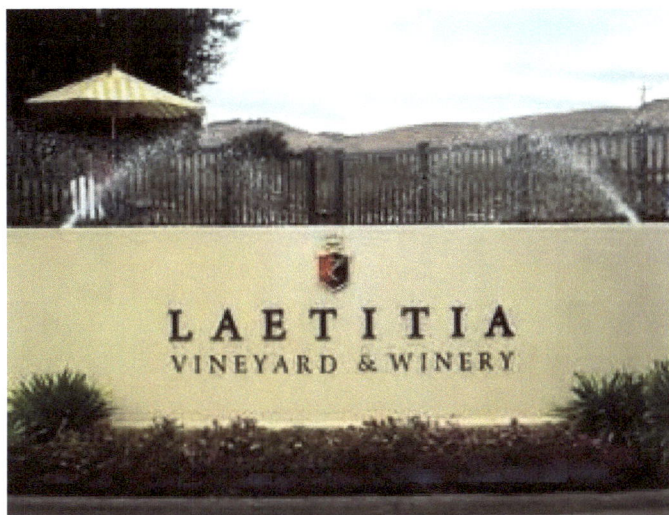

Since 1982, "Laetitia" Vineyard and Winery has produced elegant wines that champion the exceptional character and diversity of the Arroyo Grande Valley in Coastal California. Originally founded by an established French Champagne House from Epernay, the Laetitia estate carries on in the longstanding traditions of Burgundy and Champagne with a focus on an outstanding elaboration of Pinot Noirs and sparkling wines. Valuing legacy, balance, innovation and sustainable practices from harvest to glass, the "Laetitia" team works meticulously from vintage to vintage to ensure that every bottle is as expressive as the land from which it originates.

Far from the windswept coastal hills, a "sister" company lies on a land of elevated, quiet grace. Framed by chalky cliffs and planted to vines that are drenched in sun by day and chilled by the cover of night. This is the Santa Barbara Highlands Vineyard, the home of "Nadia" wines, crowning the high-elevation *terroir* and inexhaustible potential of the Sierra Madre. *Bordeaux* and *Rhone* variety grapes espress eloquently its wines. This are the jewels of the large collection where the Pinot Noir is King.

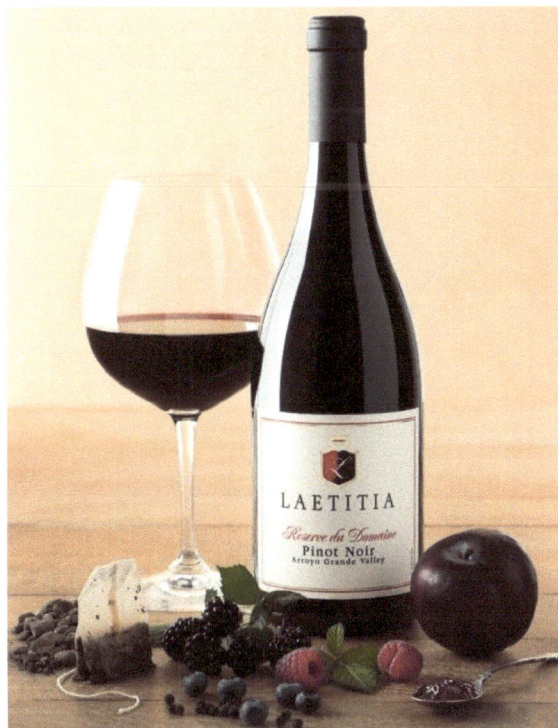

"LAETITIA" finest:

'12 Estate Pinot Noir – A seductive nose reminiscent of ripe plum and blackberry,
with layered components of earth, violets and Asian spice. The palate reveals supple tannins and lively acids accented with pretty hints of *framboise* and underlying notes of dark chocolate and rye. Try with caramelized onion and goat cheese *crostinis,* smoked pork, poultry and all game.

'12 Reserve Pinot Noir – A rich plum hue and intense candied cherry, leather, white pepper and true Cuban-cigar box aromas mark the 2012 vintage of this wine. The thick bouquet lingers and continues on to the palate with complex layers of black fruits, rich mocha and baking spice lingering to an intense finish. Great with BBQ meats, lamb and hard cheeses.

87

'12 Whole Cluster – This wine is marked by a refreshing grip in mouth feel and a singular focus on the palate. Crisp notes of cassis, whole-leaf tobacco and black peppercorn overwhelm the senses, while a touch of sweet oak and sultry black tea round out the profile beautifully. Look to pair with roasted duck, lean meats and caramelized carrots.

"NADIA"'s best:

'13 Sauvignon Blanc – Mango peel aromas waft from the glass weaving through a redolence of tropical kiwi and night blooming jasmine. On the palate, cooked stone fruit and zingy key lime notes are softened by hints of dried field grass. A refreshing mineral-driven backbone is balanced by weight and texture imparted by 15% aging in neutral French oak, while the remainder aged in stainless steel. Perfect with seafood and white fish. Great for a festive "copeo".

'12 Cabernet Sauvignon – Wild blackberry and forest floor notes enthusiastically emerge from the glass as sweet cigar smoke and perfumed violet weave throughout Layers of chocolate covered cherries, anise and salty sea air are underscore by rich cedar with firm, yet supple tannin unwinding through time in the glass. Look to pair with a bison burger topped with sautéed mushrooms. Great also with most grilled red meats.

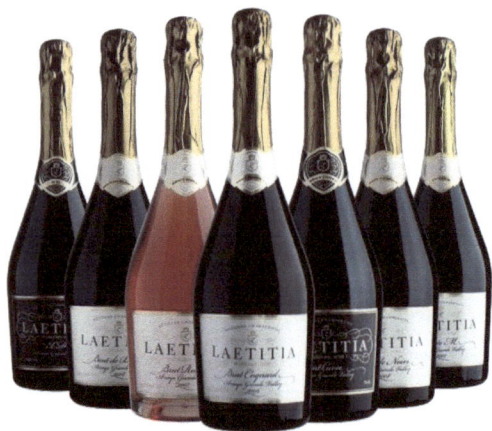

SPARKLING:

"Laetitia" Brut Cuvée N/V – Gala apple, streams of bubbles and soft melon notes meet to create this festive sparkling wine comprised of Pinot Noir, Chardonnay and Pinot Blanc varieties espectively.
Lemon chiffon and sultry pear framed by freshly baked "challah" bread come forward on second approach of our House Sparkling Wine, great for all celebrations, pairing with most dishes and Oriental cuisine.

2011 "Laetitia" Brut Rosé – Beautifully blush in color with glints of copper throughout the streams of tiny bubbles, our famous Brut Rosé is an attention grabber. On the palate, freshly-pick strawberries, tart watermelon rind and quenching acidity mark the 2011 vintage, while secondary notes of freshly baked *brioche* and baking spices speak to the balance and complexity of this very special wine.

What a great tour !

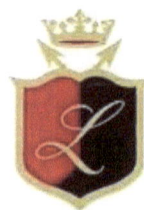

A UNIQUE COLLECTION OF THE FINEST COGNACS
Open the door of the TESSERON Home to find it

This new year I'd like to introduce you to **"Tesseron Cognac"**, the family owned Cognac House known to insiders and connoisseurs for blending some of the world's finest Grande Champagne cognacs, representing four generations and over 100 years of tradition in growing, distilling, aging and blending the finest reserve cognacs. This treasure dates back to the nineteenth century when Abel Tresseron acquired the property in *Chateauneuf-sur-Charente* and began his collection of rare and priceless cognacs.

By unveiling the two treasures of the House, "The Signature Collection" and "Royal Blend" decanters, Alfred and Melanie Tesseron, the third and fourth generations guardians of the family business, have crafted something highly desirable for cognac aficionados to covet, while preserving and nurturing, their family's traditions of blending exclusively XO cognacs (XO stands for Extra Old).

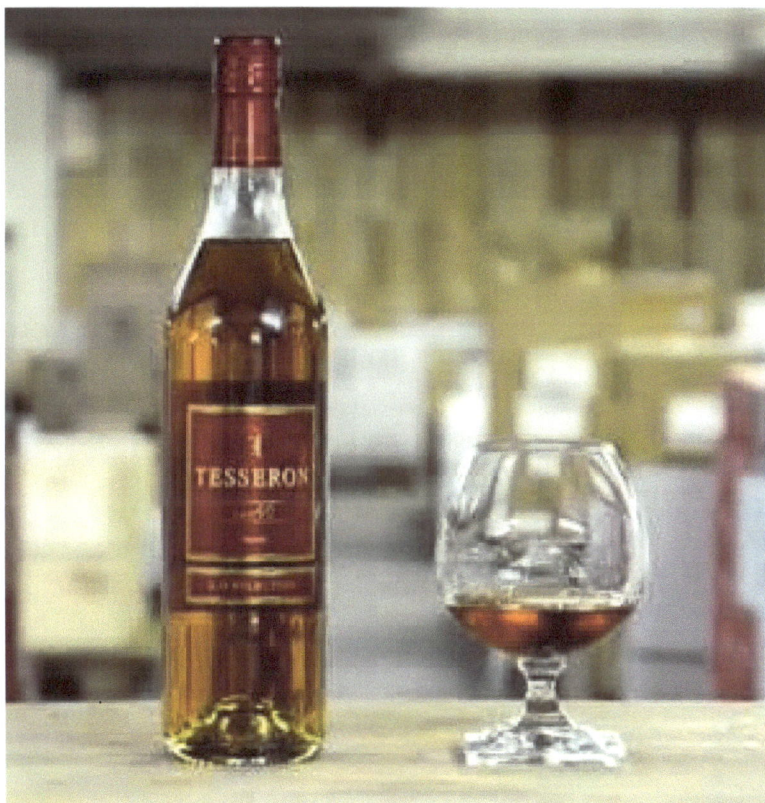

The cool, damp Tesseron cellars dating back to the XII Century were once part of the cript of the local Church. It is here where all started.

"THE SIGNATURE COLLECTION": Bottled and hand labeled on demand, pays homage to the style of cognac established by Tesseron Cognac founder Abel, who secured the family's reputation as a producer of ultimate luxury Cognac. In addition to personally blending each Cognac, Alfred designed the coffrets for the three stunning decanters, creating breathtaking showpieces that evoke images of sophistication and glamour:

XO Passion – Is an assemblage of 30 separate *eaux de vie,* each aged more than ten years and selected for their elegance, lightness and very floral quality.

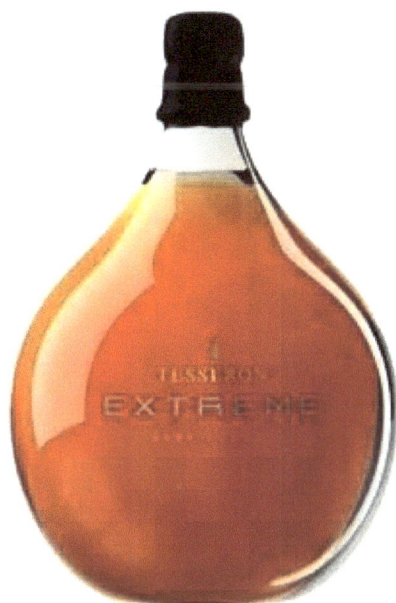

Extra LEGEND – Is a marriage of the finest reserves of Grande Champagne from 50 separate *eaux de vie,* each aged for a generation. It boasts of a beautiful maturity with notes of cooked fruits and velvety finish.

TRESOR – Is a blend of more than 100 separate *eaux de vie,* aged more than two generations in the renowned Tesseron family's *"Paradis"* cellars. It has a rich, bold character that also displays tremendous finesse and length.

"ROYAL BLEND":   Made upon request for one of the European royal families, **Royal Blend** is a tribute to the Tesseron family's expertise cultivating very old, rare cognacs.   With only 1,000 bottles produced for the world, each bottled in a decanter reminiscent of the style with which rare cognacs are aged in the Tesseron family's 12th century *"Paradis"*cellars.

Royal Blend – This is a selction of fifty distinct Grande Champagne blends from *Ugni Blanc* and *Colombard* grapes, all aged for more than two generations. Lively and vivid with exceptional fruity and floral characters, one sip transports you to the harvest in Cognac.

Nothing better to crown a festive celebration or friendly gatherings!

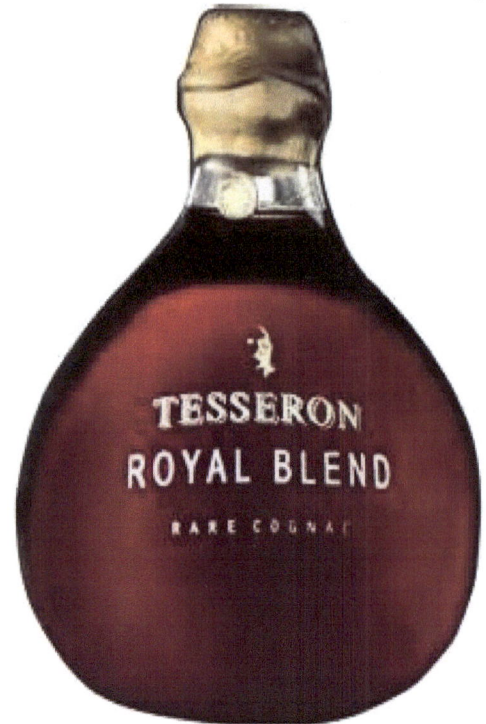

A MODEL AMERICAN WINERY

"Newton". High elevation fruit in an ideal hillside property of Napa Valley

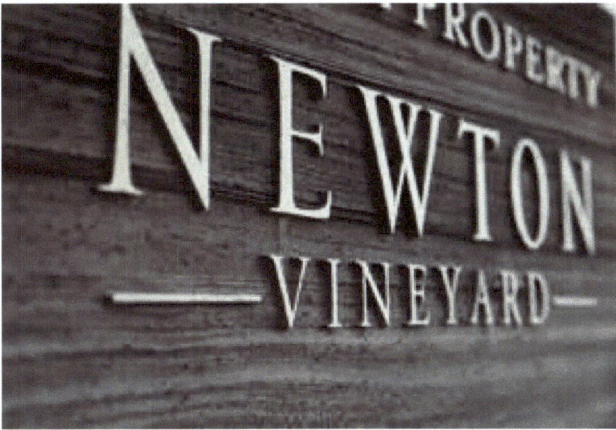

The founders of "Newton Vineyards", Su Hua and Peter Newton, believed in the quality, character and rich flavors of higher elevation vineyards, so they set out to find the ideal hillside property for planting grapes. They found it in 1977 on Spring Mountain, where they purchased one square mile of tumbling slopes overlooking Napa Valley, the California grape kingdom. The Newtons were among the first to recognize the area as a prime viticultural region. The vineyard is planted on 560 acres at elevations ranging from 500 to 1,600 feet above the sea level. The terraced vineyards provide varying sun exposure and contain diverse soil types that allow for several *Bordeaux* varietals to thrive, including Merlot, Cabernet Franc, Cabernet Sauvignon and Petit Verdot. Their Chardonnay is grown in Carneros, on the gentle rolling hills that border San Pabl Bay. Its breezes and morning fog combine to create an ideal microclimate for Chardonnay.

The estate, designed by Su Hua Newton, reflects the tastes and heritage of its founders. A formal English parterre garden reflects the birthplace of Peter Newton.
The Chinese red gate, striking cedar pagoda and other Asian accents reveal the culture of his wife Su Hua. Wine caves are burrowed into the hillside and the fermentation room is subtly hidden by the gardens, intermingling with the natural surroundings. The vineyard parcels themselves are carefully scattered among the forested land to maintain a balance with the native habitat.

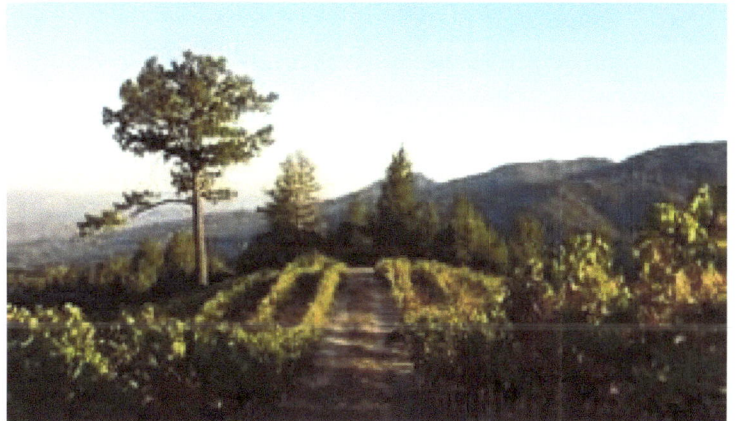

Newton wines are naturally fermented using indigenous yeast to preserve the natural fruit characteristics achieved in the vineyard. The winery was custom designed to ferment its blocks separately, preserving the individualism of each parcel. These subtle variances, when blended together, contribute to the overall complexity of the finished wine. Newton Vineyards is well known for its "Unfiltered" wines, bottled without filtration to preserve the integrity and natural essence of superior fruit and to foster the resulting wines unique aroma and flavor. The outcome of working in tandem with Nature is a range of wines considered among the finest in existence.

Newton presents the three top and most popular wines of the collection:

2012 Unfiltered Chardonnay – VINIFICATION: This is a 100% barrel-fermented wine, using indigenous yeasts. The wine is then aged for a total of 15 months in French oak barrels. TASTING NOTES: The warm 2012 vintage resulted in a complex, rich and powerful Chardonnay with aromas of jasmine, apricot, grapefruit and subtle spice. The palate is fresh with a creamy texture marked by notes of pear and roasted almonds.

FOOD PAIRING: With its benchmark balance of fruit and acidity, this Unfiltered Chardonnay is delicious with a wide range of dishes, from roasted sea bass to pasta in a butter sauce. It makes a lovely aperitif served with *crostinis* topped with wild mushrooms or truffle-flavored popcorn, ideal wine for a first course with lobster bisque, oysters, and a memorable wine for a cheese course.

2012 Unfiltered Merlot – VINIFICATION: Once harvested, the Merlot grapes are sorted inspecting individual berries to ensure uniform, perfect ripeness. The juice then undergoes 3 to 5 days of a cold soak followed by 8 to 10 days of fermentation using native yeasts. The wine then rested on the skins for a week longer to develop additional complexity. TASTING NOTES: The aromas of this delectable Merlot are redolent of ripe blueberries and Satsuma plums with hints of violet, mocha, mint and savory black fruit flavors. It is richly textured with a firm structure. The long finish is round and warm with toasted cedar, mocha and roasted coffee beans flavors. FOOD PAIRING: The 2012 Merlot is a robust wine that can be enjoyed with a wide range of dishes, from red wine-braised lamb to grilled salmon. It is extremely versatile complementing with rich vegetarian dishes, such as lentils in a *curry* sauce or mushrooms and parmesan tart.

2012 Unfiltered Cabernet Sauvignon – VINIFICATION: Following the same initial procedure we apply to the Unfiltered Merlot, this wine also rested on the skins for a week longer for a higher complexity. Finally is pressed and aged for 16 months in 40% French oak barrels. TASTING NOTES: Aromas of Dutch cocoa, mulberry, vanilla and herb-infused tapenade lead to a rich and full plush palate. Flavors of mocha, cassis and cedar are complemented by a slightly chalky, but fine, long finish. FOOD PAIRING: This wine is a sublime representation of the 2012 vintage with bold flavors that demand a meal of equal stature. Consider pairing this wine with roasted or braised beef dishes, pasta with rich tomato-based sauces or grilled lamb with a savory rub.

A vivid example for all wineries!

"SALTON" THE UNIQUE WINES OF BRAZIL

A life, four generations

Telling the story of a family is always something fascinating, especially when this story revolves around the drink of the gods – WINE. *"Salton"* is the oldest, still operating winery in Brazil. Its history dates back to 1878 when Antonio Domenico Salton, an amateur-winemaker, emigrated from Italy to Brazil in hopes of new opportunities. *Paul Salton officially established Vinicola Salton in 1910* along with his brothers.

While they ran the business facing hard times, the second generation of the Salton family gradually started to take over, also encountering many difficulties and facing major crises. They were at risk of closing their doors, but they did not give up, transforming the company as needs arose. Amid times of trouble, there were great achievements.

It was time for the third generation to also enter the company and work in different departments. Is very important to highlight the work carried out by Angelo Salton, who was a true Public Relations officer at *Vinicola Salton* and during the time, he ran the company he promoted its products, showed its potential and positioned *Salton* among the largest wineries in the world.

Currently, the fourth generation is involved in seeking new improvements and the promotion of Vinicola *Salton* image. This generation is also focused on main-taining traditions combined with the importance of innovation and technological development. Today the Winery is a benchmark in the Brazilian Industry in terms of innovation, modernization of processes, winemaking controls, organization and hygiene. Presenting today's most popular wines.

SALTON INTENSO: Cabernet Franc 2013 – Tannat 2013 – Sparkling Brut. Sparkling Traditional Method – Moscato Bubbles – Sweet White Sparkling.
SALTON CLASSIC: Cabernet Sauvignon – Cabernet Franc – Merlot – Tannat – Chardonnay – Riesling.
SALTON LUNAE FRISANTE: Cabernet Sauvignon and Merlot – Lunae Branco Moscato – Lunae Rosé Demi-Sec.
SALTON FLOWERS: Demi- Sec White Wine – Dry White Wine – Dry Red Wine – Sweet Red Wine.
SALTON TALENTO: Dry Red & Dry White Wines.

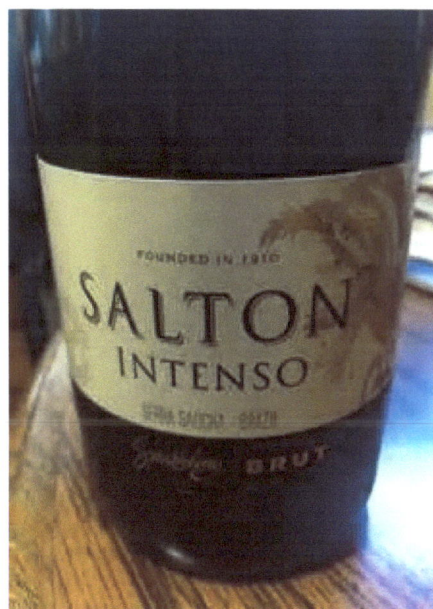

Let's drink'm all in Ipanema!

BRANDY DE JEREZ

The evocative Grand Spirit from Spain and its unique Solera ageing method

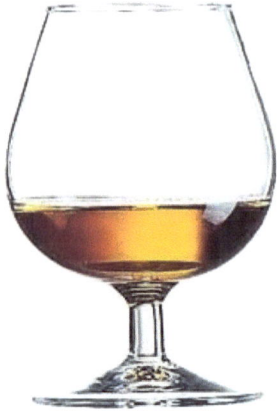

Brandy is the first most elegant distilled spirit in History. The art of "distillation" was known to the East long before it was introduced into the West. It was used by the earliest experimentalists. The father of metaphysics, Aristotle, mentioned that pure water can be made by the evaporation of sea water and Pliny the Elder, the illustrious historian, described a primitive method of condensation activated by heat generated by stills. However, the Arabians improved the apparatus creating the "alembic", or pot still, a water cooling system, principle of the modern industrial distillation. Fruits, roots and plants were utilized as the basic ingredients, resulting in the production of a powerful spirit named by the Arabians "alcohol". The Moors introduced the process into Spain, founding their Empire's capital in Andalucía, making of this region the lush fertile garden of Occidental Europe. By the 13th century the craft of alcoholic distillation had already travel to Italy and France were the resulting finished product was named eau-de-vie ("water of life") due to its curative, aphrodisiac and light minding proprieties.

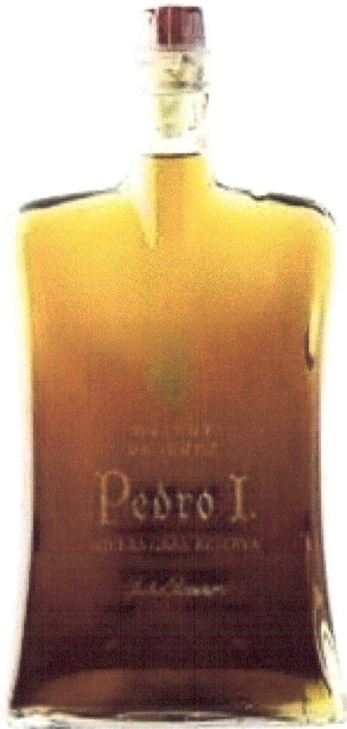

Brandewijn ("burnt wine"), was the Dutch denomination for a new style of *"water of life"* which was soon shorten by the English merchants as "brandy".

There are only three official brandy regions in the world. Cognac and Armagnac in France and Jerez in Andalucía, southwestern Spain. A region where the rich, chalky soil and a climate affected by both, the Atlantic and the Mediterranean, create a unique atmosphere conducive for producing some of the best sherries and brandies in the world. The wine producers of Jerez have made regulations controlling the

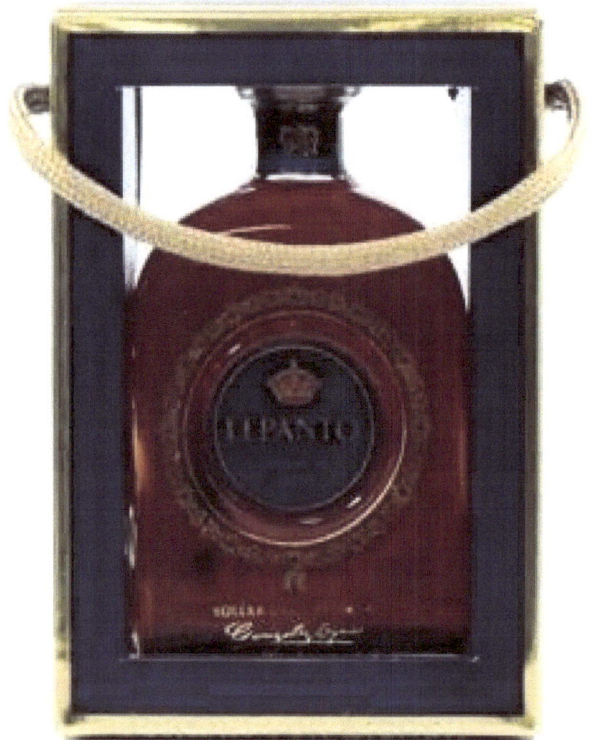

94

production process of their wines and spirits dating back to the XV century. It was 1891 the year in which "The Jerez Denomination of Origin" (DO) was finally ratified internationally.

T his DO is closely controlled by a *Consejo Regulador* (regulatory council) to ensure that strict production and ageing processes are adhere to, checking their every aspect, from the vineyards to harvesting procedures, to ageing and quality control. *Brandy de Jerez* requires a mandatory following of the *Solera* ageing method, a clockwork system in which time, transfers and gravity are involved as the chart presented in this article explains. The Spanish word *solera* derives from *suelo* ("floor" in English) due to the ground alignment of the barrels ready to be bottled. Is also a synonym for "lineage" or "great tradition" in the Spanish Language.

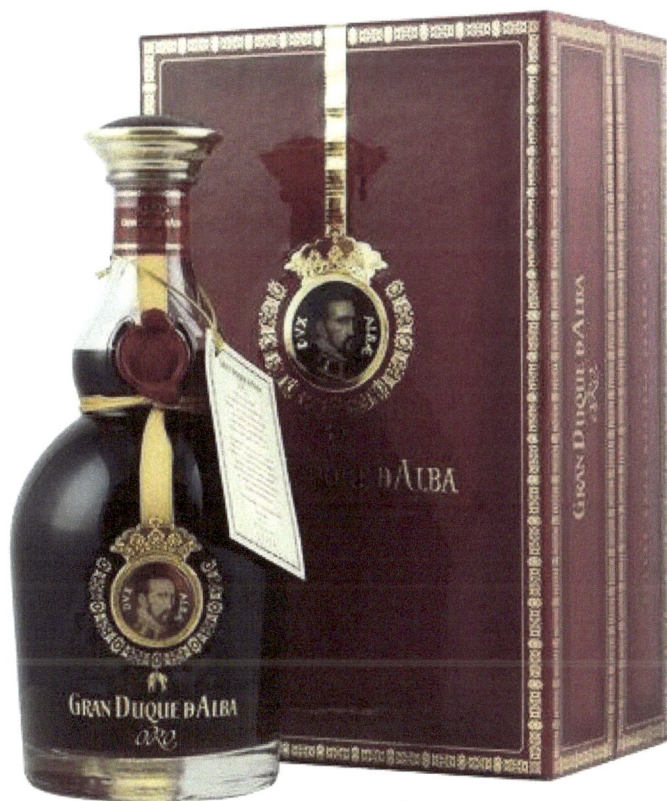

We find three different denominations in this style of brandy: *Solera* – with a minimum of three months in the cask – *Solera Reserva* after one year – *Solera Gran Reserva* requiring at least three years at rest before bottling. Is best served at room temperature in a snifter during dessert or at coffee time. It also can be enjoyed neat as a digestive or in a variety of cocktails.

Let's elaborate on the finest Premium Brandies *Solera Gran Reserva* of Jerez in the international market:

GRAN DUQUE DE ALBA: This rich, super-premium brandy has been aged for 12 years in oak casks that previously held *oloroso* sherry. Like its namesake, the Grand Duke of the regiment of Flanders and Viceroy of the Low Countries, this is a bold, aristocratic brandy with an impeccable heritage produced by the world-renowned Williams & Humpert bodega in Jerez. Light mahogany in color with gold reflections offers undertones of roasted nuts, warm caramel and dark fruit notes tinged with brown spice. The finish is long and satisfying with a soft after-taste.

 GRAN DUQUE DE ALBA ORO: An ultra-premium Gran Reserva Especial aged for a minimum of 25 years through seven separate *soleras*.

CONDE DE OSBORNE: The House of Osborne, headquartered in *El Puerto de Santamaría* – adjacent to Jerez – was founded in 1772 and is one of the oldest firms of wine and spirits producers in Spain. This elegant brandy *Solera Gran Reserva* has been aged for a minimum of 10 years using barrels that once housed sweet Pedro Ximénez sherry. With a polish mahogany captivating color, Conde de Osborne's heady aroma reveals oak wood, sweet cacao, smooth vanilla and the fruity warmth of dried plums and raisins. With a silky honeyed flavor, it also develops a hint of citrus complementing its chocolate after-taste and persistent finish.

SALVADOR DALI Collector's Bottle Limited-Edition: For the introduction of its top of the line *Solera Gran Reserva* in 1964, the House of Osborne commissioned none other than the inimitable Salvador Dalí to design a bottle and label that would be utterly original and deserving of the exquisite aristocratic elixir it would house. The result is a singular creation of an unconventional milk-white bottle and the artist's personal interpretation of the Osborne family crest, enveloping a magnificent blend of the oldest *soleras* of their bodegas.

LEPANTO BRANDY DE JEREZ: This masterpiece is named to commemorate the XVI century naval battle where Spain defeated the Ottoman Empire's fleet. *Lepanto* is victorious as well in the battle of premium brandies. Its refined taste and rich character match the unique and colorful history of its Spanish homeland. González Byass Co., producers of *Lepanto* and some of the finest sherries and brandies in the world, was founded by Manuel María González Angel in 1835 and still in hands of the founding family.

The *Solera Gran Reserva* of *Lepanto Brandy de Jerez* was born in 1896. Produced from Palomino grapes, the spirit is twice distilled, a process requiring constant attention and great expertise. Matured in barrels previously used for Fino sherry production and aged for a minimum of 15 years, *Lepanto* presents a topaz color sprinkled with Spanish gold hues. Smoky aromas of vanilla, nut, oily leather and hot pepper lead to a wide array of flavors such as caramel, vanilla, dried almonds and raisins offering a long woody finish.

CARDENAL MENDOZA SOLERA GRAN RESERVA: Now, over 200 years old, Sánchez Romate Hermanos is one of the oldest and more respected bodegas in Spain. In 1887, its owners began to make a unique brandy for their own consumption. The four original casks in which this brandy was aged are still carefully preserved as a much-treasured relic. As a result of its exceptionally high quality, it gained great fame and the winery decided to market it with the name of *Cardenal Mendoza*, paying tribute to Pedro González de Mendoza, Cardinal of The Holly See and a historical figure who played a crucial role in the conquest of the Muslim kingdom of Granada and specially in the discovery of America, as he interceded on behalf of Christopher

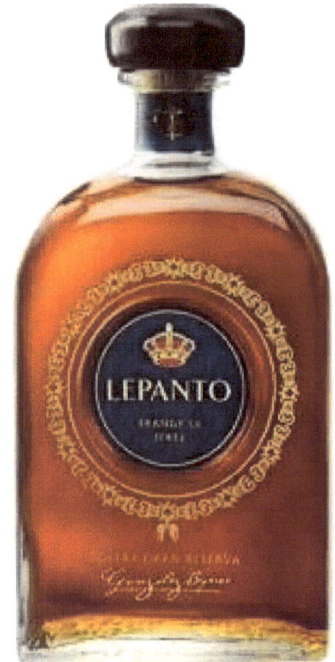

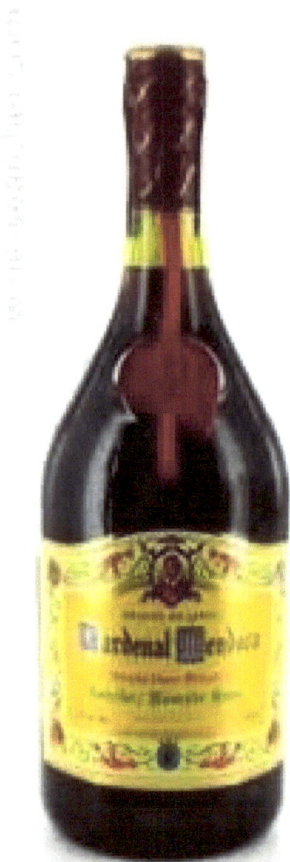

Columbus's project before the Catholic Monarchs. In today's market, *Cardenal Mendoza* presents three different versions of this eminent spirit:

"Clásico": Bright, transparent, dark mahogany colours. With an average age of 15 years in american oak casks pre-treated with Oloroso and Pedro Ximénez sherry, offers a round, clean, elegant, wine-like aromas.

Long, warm and balanced on the palate with no harsh edges and a harmony of subtle flavors with an intense finish of raisins and plumps.

"Carta Real": It needs a minimum of 30 years to carry its name. Carta Real reveals itself as a seductive brandy with bright hues of old mahogany. Its elegant aromas of old wood with hints of sweet raisins and plumps along with superbly round and persistent flavors are this brandy's exceptional characteristics, grown both in intensity and subtlety over time.

"Non Plus Ultra": In 1971, shortly before the bicentennial of Sánchez Romate Hermanos, 38 casks of *Cardenal Mendoza* were reserved to celebrate the event. This limited "reserva" gave birth to "Non Plus Ultra", an inimitable brandy with an average age of 50 years, of dark mahogany color, sleek and exciting. The traditional aromas of raisins and plumps, reminiscent of Oloroso sherry, persist intensely while showing a dry and delicate performance on the palate with a long velvety after-taste of nutmeg and dried orange Spirit of "España", Star of "Jerez".

Enjoy them all. Have a sip of History!

WHISKY, THE *ACQUA VITAE* OF SCOTLAND

Enjoyed for over five hundred years, is today the most popular spirit in the Planet

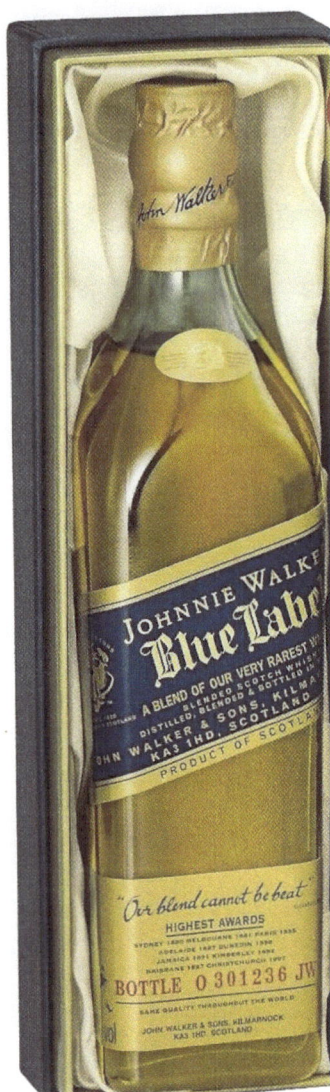

Whisky is an alcoholic beverage obtained from the distillation of a fermented blend of mashed cereal grains or of a single barley malt, suitably aged in wood, usually white oak. It is "whisky" in Scotland and Canada and "whiskey" in Ireland and the U.S. There is no precise record of when whisky was first distilled in either Scotland or Ireland. Its name evolved from the Scots Celtic word *uisgebeatha* translation of the Latin term *aqua vitae*, the water of life, which eventually was shorten and anglicized into "whisky" in the XVII century. The earliest direct account is found in the Scottish Exchequer records of 1494, which lists: "Eight bolls of malt for Friar John wherewith to make *aqua vitae*". There must have been knowledge of the art long before, since Al-Bukassen, the Arabian alchemist, had described the distillation process in his writings of the X century. The whiskies produced in each country are distinctive in character due to the difference in method of production, type of grains utilized and, most important, the quality and proprieties of the water employed. Only in Scotland can be found the spring water that rises

through a red granite formation and then passes through peat moss country, the base of this inimitable product. Scotch whisky is a weird paradox of a drink. It is made from a few, very humble ingredients and yet is infinitely varied and often of an incredible complexity. Diluted in a splash of pure water is the ideal method of consumption. It soothes away stress one moment and fires up passion the next. It is a beguiling temptress that allows one early sip to slip smoothly into another by night, only to turn into the most vicious demon in the morning, managing somehow to capture a little of the bitter-sweet melancholic beauty of the place. It is Scotland in a bottle.

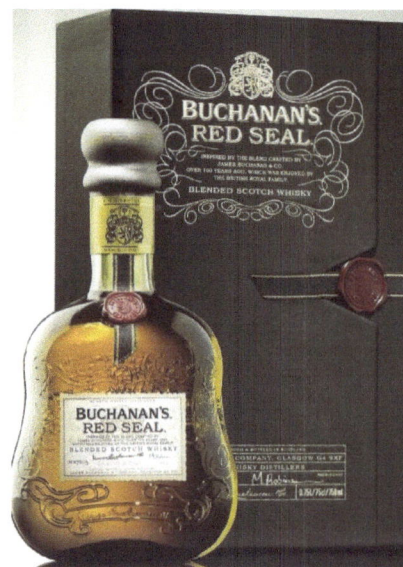

In the international market, this elixir appears with bold bottle designs and a variety of ages. Let's comment on some of its top ambassadors:

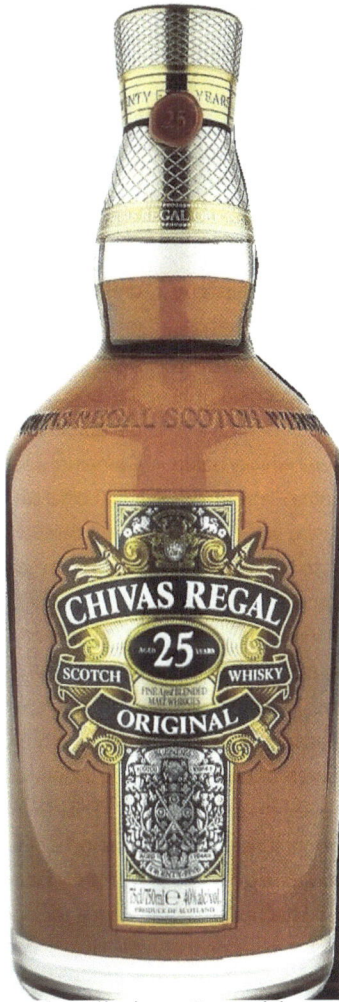

JOHNNIE WALKER: Back in 1820 when our hero was parading around his native Kilmarnok in top hat and tails, he was actually just 15. He had recently inherited 417 sterling pounds from his father which was to be held in trust until he was old enough to open a grocery shop in the town. Time later he taught his son Alexander tea and malt blending, but there is no documentation of whisky making until "The Spirits Act"was born in 1860, allowing blended scotch to take off. The business began to grow and by the mid-1860s the firm was selling 100,000 gallons of whisky at year in Glasgow and beyond. The world-famous logo of the young dandy in mid-stride was sketched on the back of a menu in a London restaurant in 1908 by Tom Brown, a well known cartoonist and commercial artist. Alexander registered initially his firm as "Walker's Old Highland Whisky", but the name "Johnnie Walker" didn't appeared until 1908 launched as **Black Label** 12 yr. Old", the most popular today. **Red Label** (8yr.) and **Gold Label** (18 yr.) are also part of the family, however the patriarch is the 25 year old **Blue Label**, created from a blend of the rarest and most expensive whiskies in the world. The nose has hints of smoke, sherry and fruitcake; the body is soft and mellow with *jerez oloroso*, honey and vanilla notes and dark chocolate overtones.

CHIVAS REGAL: The world's first luxurious whisky was created through the unique combination of skill, heritage and precious stocks of superb quality malt whiskies. It was brothers James and John Chivas, true pioneers of the art of blending, the followers of two fundamental principles: the use of old, mature stocks and a distinct Spayside accent, a region blessed with pristine water, fresh air and rich barley fields. The Chivas brothers had the foresight to invest in the Strathisla Distillery, the oldest in the Highlands, been in the 1890s when they culminated into the final masterpiece that today is the outstanding Chivas Regal blend. In 1923 the Chivas Brothers received a royal recognition by becoming "Purveyor of Scotch Whisky to His Majesty King George V ". This aristocratic collection presents a 12 year old, **The Original**; the 18 year old bottle bearing the **Signature** of Colin Scott, master distiller of the House, offering his personal blend of stocks reserved exclusively to bring depth and add exceptional richness. But the greatest news were the arrival to the shelves in 2007 of the latest creation, **Chivas Regal 25** year old. Perfectly balanced and immeasurably smooth, with aromas of stone fruit leading to complex notes of creamy marzipan, nuts and chocolate-orange, extended to a luxuriously rounded finish. "It is the quintessential Chivas Regal" affirms Scott.

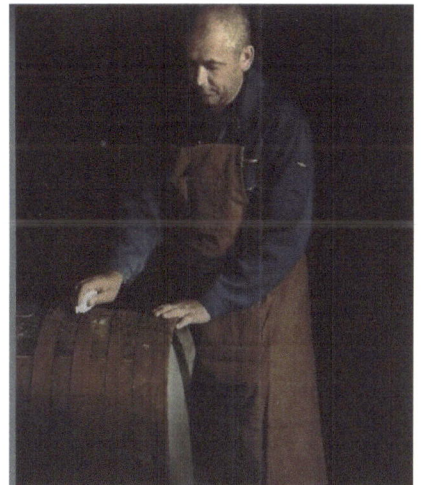

BUCHANAN'S: Born in 1849 to Scottish emigrants, James Buchanan started his whisky business without capital or experience. When he was 30, he became a London agent for a well-known firm in the whisky trade and he had the vision that London – and indeed the rest of England – was an untapped market for bottled Scotch Whisky leaving aside the old fashion casks. He started his own company with capital loaned to him by a good business acquaintance. By 1889 Buchanan, an innovator promoting his brand with smart advertising, had achieved great success all over Europe, winning a gold medal at the Paris Exhibition in open competition for blended scotch. While building his business and his wealth during the Victorian period he never forgot his humble beginnings, becoming a dedicated philanthropist, donating large amounts of cash to universities and hospitals and upon his death, left a considerable portion of his fortune to his devoted staff. Here is hism legacy: **Buchanan's De Luxe** (12 yrs**.), Buchanan's Super De Luxe** (18 yrs.) a gorgeous whisky with a long, full-flavoured finish and the jewel of his collection, **Red Seal** (25 yrs.) a full-bodied, richly satisfying blend with floral, fruity notes and hints of lavender, fresh green apples, oak and vanilla. Some smoky, clean sherry and lively spice tones accompany its long warm and pleasing finish.

DEWAR'S: There was no greater whisky baron than Tommy Dewar, the son of a small-time blender from Perth in the Highlands, who was sent to London in 1885 aged 21 to "wake up the south" by his father John, founder of the dynasty. While Tom played the witty front man, his brother John was the shrewd Scot who ran the production end of the business in Perth. Tommy Dewar was a consummated salesman who, in 1886 alone traveled globally visiting 26 countries while orders were successfully pouring in. He understood the power of advertising better than almost any of his contemporaries. Long before Coca-Cola discovered how to use neon to its advantage, Tommy Dewar had attached a 200 foot Scotsman to the side of a vacant tower on the south bank of the Thames river. Londoners were stunned by this giant Highlander, made of hundreds of light bulbs, whose kilt appeared to sway in the breeze as his right hand repeatedly raised a glass of Dewar's White Label to his lips. The actual hero behind the scenes was Alexander Cameron, master distiller *par excellence* who joined the firm in 1890, the creator of White Label, a blend of 40 different malts that was launched at the turn of the century. By 1900 a one million gallon mark production was reached. Today **Dewar's White Label** is the most sold scotch whisky in the U.S. Recently, Dewar's released its masterpiece **Signature**, a delicate 25 year old blend of limited production, with aromas of honey, raisins and vanilla. Lightly sweet and smooth in the palate with a long slightly dry finish.

THE GLENLIVET: Revising the whole history of whisky-making in the Highlands of Scotland the word "Glenlivet" captures the very spirit of defiance of the law. Fiscally undeclared domestic "moon shine"- making under "whisky" appellation was rampant. The story of Glenlivet begins in 1824 with George Smith, who was the first in the region to take out a license for operating a distillery at a farm leased by his father some years before. After the first year the distillery was producing a hundred gallons of single malt whisky at week, but George couldn't compete with the organized contraband surrounding his land. Since most Scots and English preferred illicit whisky, the smugglers were looked on benignly and seen as romantic figures. However, by 1834 the battle against the illegal trade was won, and Smith's Glenlivet prospered and spread to Aberdeen, Perth and the seaport of Leith. He was also

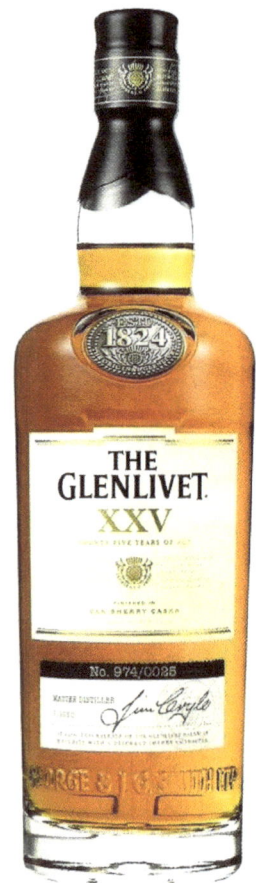

supplying malt whisky to Andrew Usher, the father of blended Scotch, who launched "Old Vatted Glenlivet" in the mid-nineteen century. When George Smith died rich in 1871, Glenlivet had become the best known distillery in Scotland. The stories of smugglers and piracy, true most of them and passed on to generations, was the best publicity for this legendary scotch. And George Smith knew it. This single malt is largely varied: **The Glenlivet** (12 yrs.); **French Oak Reserve** (15 yrs.); **The Glenlivet Nadurra** (min. 16 yrs.); **The 18 Year Old**; **Archive 21 Year Old**. The firm is highly proud of the recent release of **The Glenlivet XXV** (25 yrs.) made from a 1980 vintage selection with intense and deep sherry notes of fruit and spices accompanied by sandalwood and a touch of cedar. Hints of candied tangerines, pineapple and pralines can also be found. The taste is silky smooth and sweet releasing ginger and cinnamon before developing into dark chocolate and spicy orange peel noticeable in its dry finish.

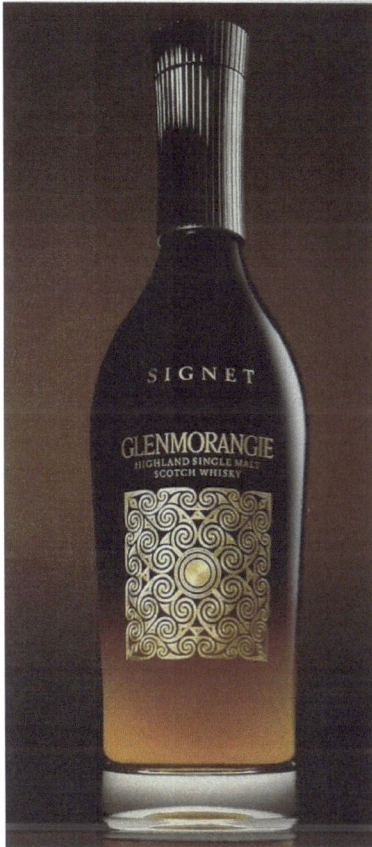

GLENMORANGIE: The distillery Glenmorangie House, one of the pioneers of Single Malt whisky, was establish in 1843 by the pre-historic Cadboll Stone dolmens surrounding the region. For the next forty years William Matheson, the original operator of the distillery, carried on in a rudimentary fashion somehow managing to produce 20.000 gallons at year by the time Alfred Barnard, the Victorian whisky writer, paid a visit in the 1880s. he described the distillery as "the most ancient and primitive we have seen". This harsh critique attracted curious outside investors in The Glenmorangie Distillery Co. Enlarged and renewed various times throughout the century, Glenmorangie produces today some of the finest and most sophisticated Highland Single Malts in the international market. **Glenmorangie 10 Year Old Original; 18 Year Old; Glenmorangie Nectar D'Or; The Lasanta; The Quinta Ruban; Glenmorangie Quarter Century 25 Year Old** (one of the most expensive in the world with a cost of $890.00); and their newest creation just released **Glenmorangie Signet,** a secret combination of the oldest and rarest whiskies Glenmorangie has ever produced from precious ingredients, including high roasted 'chocolate' malted barley for depth and intensity. The results are sublime flavours and an encompassing velvet texture long finish.

Over eighty whisky distilleries flourish in Scotland accounting for 95% of the popular blends and a 5% of the highly appreciated single malts. 88.4 million cases of Scotch Whisky were last sold in the world, which lined up back to back will cover 17,036 miles, twice the distance between Edinburgh and Hong Kong and, as a trivial concept, 31 bottles per second are sold today out of Scotland in almost 200 global markets.

THE WINES "de lla Bellisima Italia"
Introduction and basic knowledge of this great industry

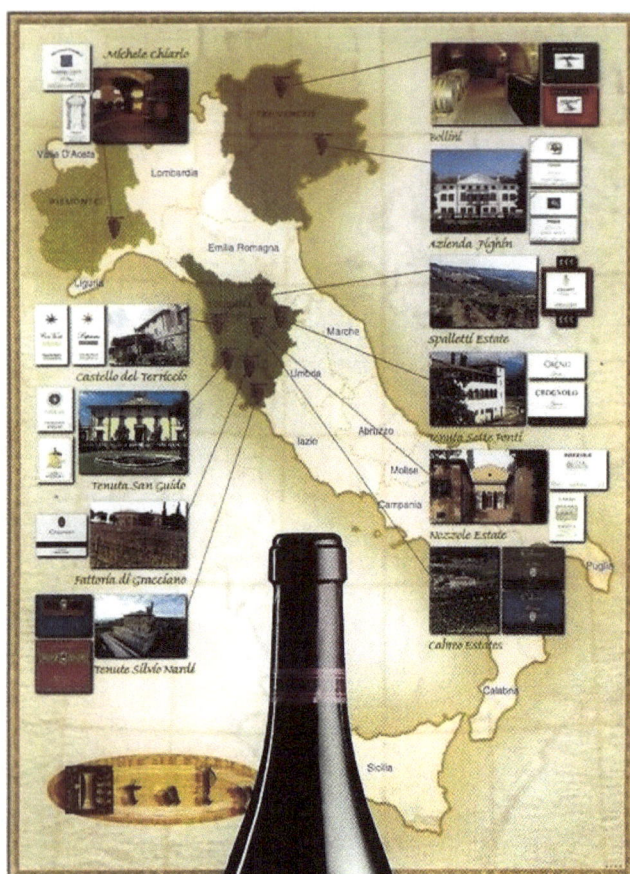

Some of the most illustrious wine estates of Italy

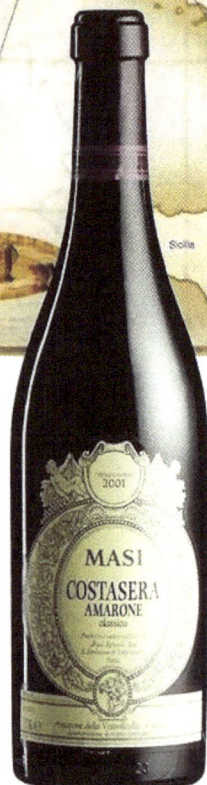

Not only is Italy the number one wine-producing country in the world today, it is also one of the oldest producers. Recent archeological finds have shown that the vine was first systematically cultivated in Italy by the Etruscans in the 8th century B.C. We can assume that efforts were made even earlier though clear proof of this has not yet been established. With the advent of the Roman Empire, advanced skills and expertise in viticulture and winemaking spread throughout Western and Central Europe. The Romans were also responsible for the development of the wine trade into a very profitable economic activity. However, with the fall of its political dominance in 476 A.D., the Empire collapsed and the peace and social tranquility vanished, not allowing the progress of viticulture. Wine growing, production and particularly the creation of fine wines declined, opening the market doors to Bordeaux, Burgundy, the Rhine and the Danube dominions.

While the Italian bankers and traders profited from wine imports, vine cultivation survived only in the form of subsistence activity among the – mainly extremely poor – rural population. Thanks to some of the most prestigious names which are still well known today in the world of Wine, such as the Antinoris and Frescobaldis and the help of the Church through local monasteries, viticulture tradition was sustained. This decline lasted into the 19th century when a new beginning emerged in Piedmont and Tuscany. Vine varieties such as Barolo, Brunello and Chianti were developed with the active involvement of French enologists. Within 150 years these wines were among the most popular and best in the world. The rest is history. To the day Italy produces wine everywhere in its soil, with the exception of some inhospitable rugged terrains. Rules and regulations were enacted for the preservation and future creation of Wine: D.O.C. (*Denominazione di Origine Contrllata*) and for the finer wines D.O.C.G. (*Denominazione di Origine Contollata e Garantita*). Labels have to express these procedence by law. Mentioning the most important D.O.C wines:

SOAVE – MOTEPULCIANO d'ABRUZZO – GRAVE del FRUILI – OLTREPO PAVESE – VALPOLICELLA – PIEDMONT – ALTO ADIGE – TRENTINO – PROSECCO di CONEGLIANO – TREBBIANO d'ABRUZZO – COLLI PIACENTINI and TOSCANA.
Indicating the finer D.O.C.G. wines: AMARONE – BARBARESCO – BAROLO – BRACHETTO – SUPER TUSCANS (Sassicaia, Ormelaia, Tignanello) – BRUNELLO di MONTALCINO – CARMIGNANO – CHIANTI – CHIANTI CLASSICO –FRANCIACORTA – TAURASI – TORGIANO ROSSO RISERVA – VINO NOBILE di MONTEPULCIANO.

The twelve most widely cultivated grape varieties: SANGIOVESSE (considered the Italian grape *par excellence*) – TREBBIANO – CATARATTO – BARBERA – ITALIA (table grape) – MERLOT – MONTEPULCIANO – MALVASIA – NEGROAMARO – REGINA (table grape) – PRIMITIVO – CALABRESE.
Great white wines are not easy to produce in Italy due to climatic circumstances.
However we can recommend the sparklings PROSECCO and MOSCATO, PINOT GRIGIO,
PINOT BIANCO – ORVIETTO – VERDICCHIO.

Italy is a red wine kingdom. Salute!

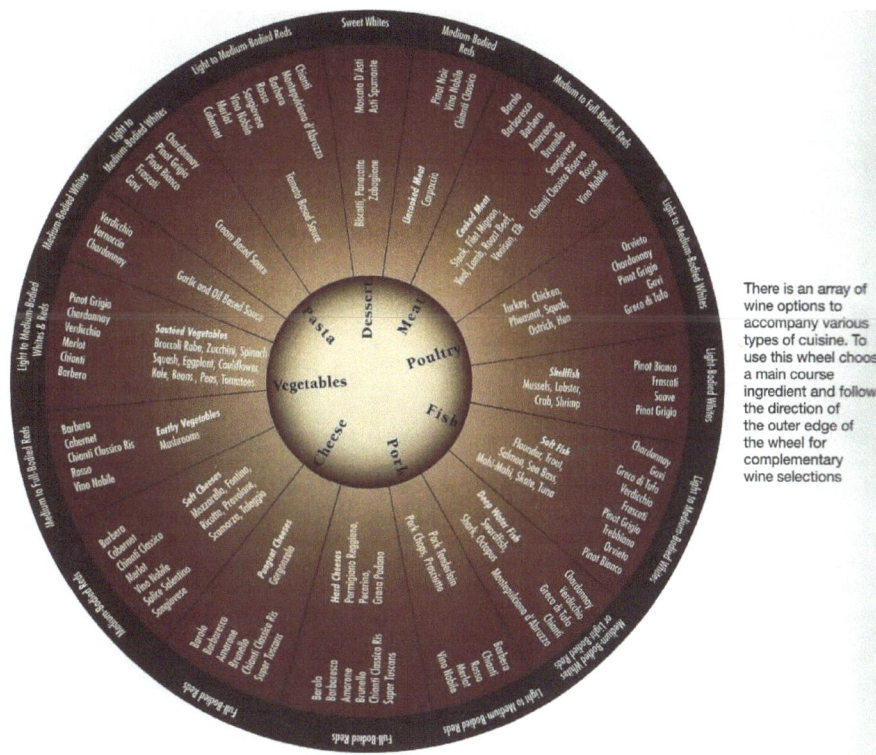

There is an array of wine options to accompany various types of cuisine. To use this wheel choose a main course ingredient and follow the direction of the outer edge of the wheel for complementary wine selections

103

NOBILITY, RICHNESS AND TRADITION
OF THE WINES OF SPAIN

Spanish wine production can be traced right back to the second millennium B.C. The Phoenicians settled in Spain around 1800 B.C. and subsequently left the first traces. The pioneering references to systematic cultivation of extensive vineyards date back to the Greek colonization of Spain. Near the Bay of Roses in the present province of Gerona, the city of Empúries was founded. Today, this quality wine-producing area of Empordá-Costa Brava is regarded as the true starting point for the spread in Spain of the Vitis vinífera, queen of all grape varieties. A few centuries later, the Roman Empire managed to industrialize wine production, distributing the wines pressed in various provinces – Catalonia, La Rioja, Aragón, and Castilla – throughout the Mediterranean region. The wines of Hispania were the favorites of the Emperors.

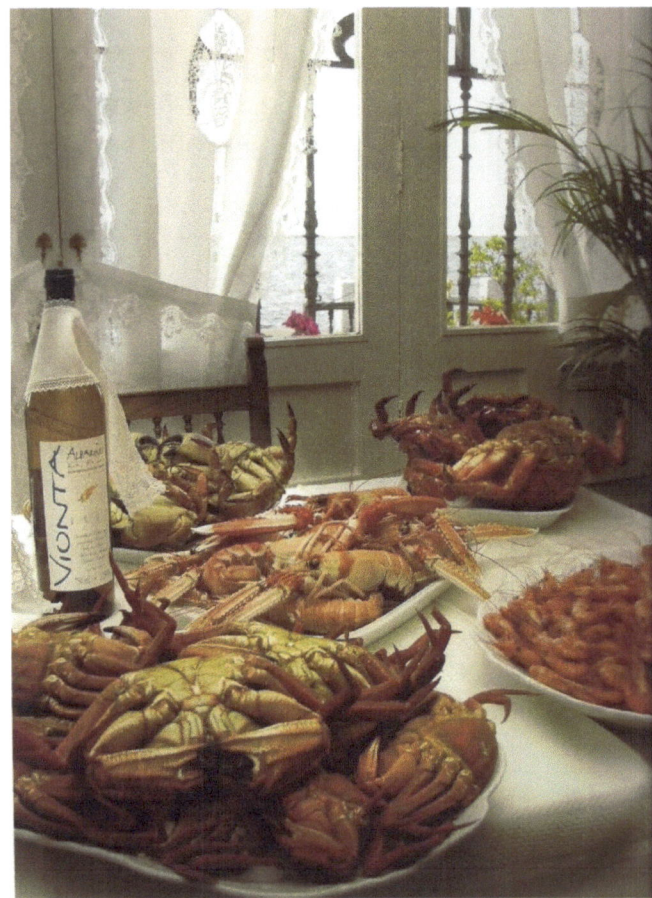

When studying Spain's wine producing you has to observe a unique point. It has the largest wine-growing area in the world, with 2.65 million acres (1.06 million ha.). 20 years ago, it was even greater at 3.75 million acres (1.5 million ha.). Contrary to the obvious assumption that nothing could be simpler than producing wine in the Spanish sunshine, the opposite has often proved to be the case. For one thing, the arid conditions in some areas and the colossal mountainous regions make intensive planting impossible. Even in many uplands of the country, and thus throughout central Spain, the sprouting vines are just as susceptible to cold and drought as any other vines. Due to these characteristics it comes as no surprise that in a country covering such a large area, the yield is comparatively low. However, regardless this climatic and geographic problems, Spain is the third wine producer in the world, currently counting with 64 Denominaciones de Origen (D.O.) and 2 Denominaciones de Origen Calificada (D.O.C.) which include La Rioja and Priorat. Most of them are technologically advanced, using updated methodology. At the same time, a younger generation of winemakers is experimenting and turning out some of the different, more modern style of wines we see coming out of Spain today.

To get a general idea, it might be helpful to have a brief look at the various climatic zones that define the country. The variety and diversity of Spanish wines is the result of the interactions of the three main zones: the Atlantic climate, the continental – four seasons weather – and the influences of the Mediterranean sea. There are also many areas of overlap, and mini-climates caused by the extremely variable terroirs of the Iberian Peninsula. The Cantabrian mountains in the north form a natural barrier that protects inland Spain from the moist Atlantic air currents; and the Sierra Morena mountain range covers the Mediterranean influence over Castile- La Mancha that runs to dominate Andalucía, creating the most favorable conditions for the birth of the unique Vino de Jerez , internationally known as Sherry, being the first Spanish wine exported since the XVI century . The must reputed wine producing regions in Spain are among many others: La Rioja, Ribera del Duero, Castilla-La Mancha, Castilla-Leon, Navarra, Aragón, Catalonia, Galicia, Andalucía, Valencia, Madrid and Extremadura. In the last 10 years Spain has added to its production the Vino Nuevo (New Wine), introducing the most creative blends in the world market. There is such a wide range of Spanish grape varieties that even high caliber experts find it bewildering. With an estimate of 600 types growing in the country, about 15 principal varieties can be described as truly Spanish and to account for about 75% of the total wine production.

From Catalunya comes Segura Viudas, one of Spain's artisan cavas producing premium Spanish sparkling wine

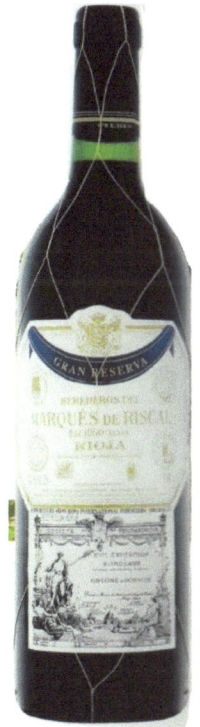

The blue-black Tempranillo grape, originally from La Rioja, is the official variety and most appreciated by the consumers, changing name by regions – Tinta del País in Ribera del Duero, Cencibel in La ancha, Ull de Llebre in Catalonia – joining Garnacha, Albariño – white – Palomino, Viura, Verdejo – these last two also white – and some of French origin such as Cabernet Sauvignon, Merlot and Syrah.

The red wine in Spain represents the favorite for the table, pairing extraordinarily with all the regional cuisines. The whites are fresh and light, ideal with seafood or simply as a copeo wine.

The sparkling wine, known as Cava, is a blend of three Catalonian grape varieties, Xarel-lo, Macabeo and Parellada original from Penedés, exclusive area for its production. For a wine to bear the Cava quality mark it must be made using the traditional method of "bottle fermentation", which is basically the french Methode Champanoise. Thus, the differences between Cava and Champagne lie in the choice of grape , soil and climatic conditions. A good Cava should be soft, fresh, have a slightly fruity-yeasty flavor and no excess of acidity.

We hope you enjoyed this tour of Spain while having a good bottle of Rioja or a glass of Fino from Jerez. Salud!

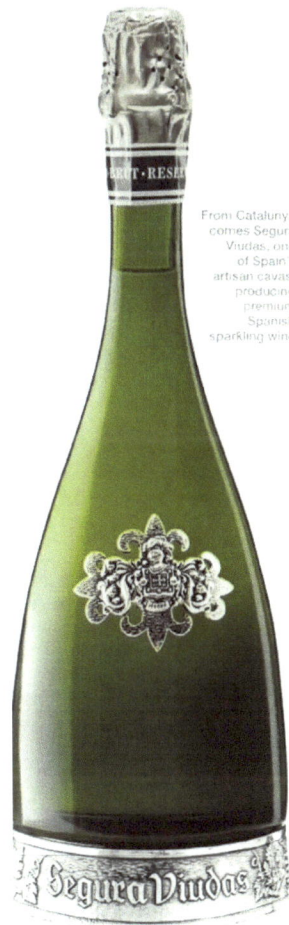

WINE AND ART
An everlasting bond

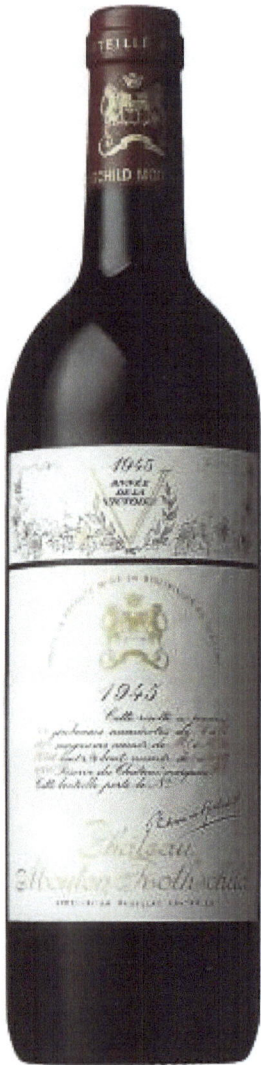

For centuries, wine has been linked to the art world ... as a matter of fact, winemaking has been referred to as a form of art by some of the most diverse civilizations in history which have left us numerous allegorical reminders of this. From Babylon and Egypt (the oldest documented vinicultures) up to today, many graphic art forms have found fascinating ways of glorifying the oldest beverage known to humanity. Since the first glass bottle emerged in England in 1708 as the universal container for wine (facilitating its packing, handling and hermetic sealing), bottle designing and label décor has become an insignia for winemakers, utilizing its artistic appearance as a powerful marketing tool. At the pinnacie of perfection in this inventive field that brings together wine making and art has stood, for many years, the Chateau Mouton Rothschild, the most prestigious Bordeaux wine of France, guided by the enthusiasm of its first owner, Baron Philippe de Rothschild, and later his daughter Baroness Philippine, who continued the tradition.

In 1924, to salute his first chateau-bottled vintage, Baron Philippe had the revolutionary idea of commissioning the poster artist Jean Carlu to design its label. Ahead of its time, this initiative did not take hold and was not repeated until 1945 when, to celebrate the end of World War 11 and the return to peace, he decided to crown the label for that year's vintage with a drawing representing the letter "V" for Victory.

From this exceptional event sprang a great tradition, and every year since, a contemporary artist has been invited to create a unique work of art for the Chateau. In the beginning, artists were somewhat reluctant to have their names linked with a consumer product, however prestigious it might've been. But fortunately, Baron Philippe's circle of friends included a number of talented master painters such as Jean Hugo, Léonor Fini and Jean Cocteau, who were swayed by his powers of persuasion.

In 1955, Georges Braque, French pioneer of the cubism art movement, agreed to iIlustrate that year's vintage and was succeeded by some of the greatest artists of our time, including Salvador Dalí, Joan Miró, Marc Chagall, Pablo Picasso, AndyWarhol, Pierre'" Soulages, Francis Bacon, Klossowski Balthus and Antoni Tapies among many others, forming a fascinating collection to which a new masterpiece is added every year.

Since 1988, when she took over the company after her father's death, Baroness Philippine de Rothschild has been responsible for choosing the featured artists and commissioning works that honor their artistic freedom while keeping in mind specific themes, such as the pleasure of drinking, the beauty of the vines and the symbol of the ram (mouton in French), which serves as the emblem for the

Chateau. Interesting enough, the artists are not paid a fee, but instead are compensated with cases of Mouton Rothschild, including of course "their" vintage.

Over the last twenty years or so, the cornmissioned works have been compiled to create a traveling exhibition, under the direction of Baroness Philippine, titled "Paintings for the Labels, " which has been shown in numerous museums throughout the world. During her reign, she has also been able to raise the star of Mouton to even higher ground. With multipliable energy, she has modernized the facilities of the family company and extended its operations to places like California and Chile, where recently, under her supervision, the Chéteeu launched Almaviva, a brand that has become the number one Cabernet Sauvignon in Latin America.

This year the firm is celebrating their latest release: the cháteau Mautan Rothschild 2006 (87% Cabernet Sauvignon -13% Merlot),which boasts a label created by German-born British painter Lucian Freud, grandson of the great Sigmund Freud, the founder of psycho analysis. His popularity is such that, in 2008, one of his artworks reached the highest sale price ever attained by a living artist to date.

With an attractive deep garnet red color, this wine reveals a complex range of aromas in which red fruit, wild blackberry and raspberry combine with spice, white pepper and vanilla to create an amazing combination that also includes some toasted notes of judicious oak.

The nose of the wine is elegant and well-structured, being further enhanced by notes of incense and jammy fruit. The attack and the roundness on the palate is prolonged by richly flavored tannins that create a creamy and powerful taste with a long and consistent finish. With a price tag of $700, it's safe to say that the Mouton Rothschild 2006 can be unanimously hailed as the most successful vintage in the Médoc region to date.

Santé!

SAINT-EMILION, THE EMBLEMATIC WINE PRIDE OF BORDEAUX

"Chateau Lassegue": Great distinction, character and elegance

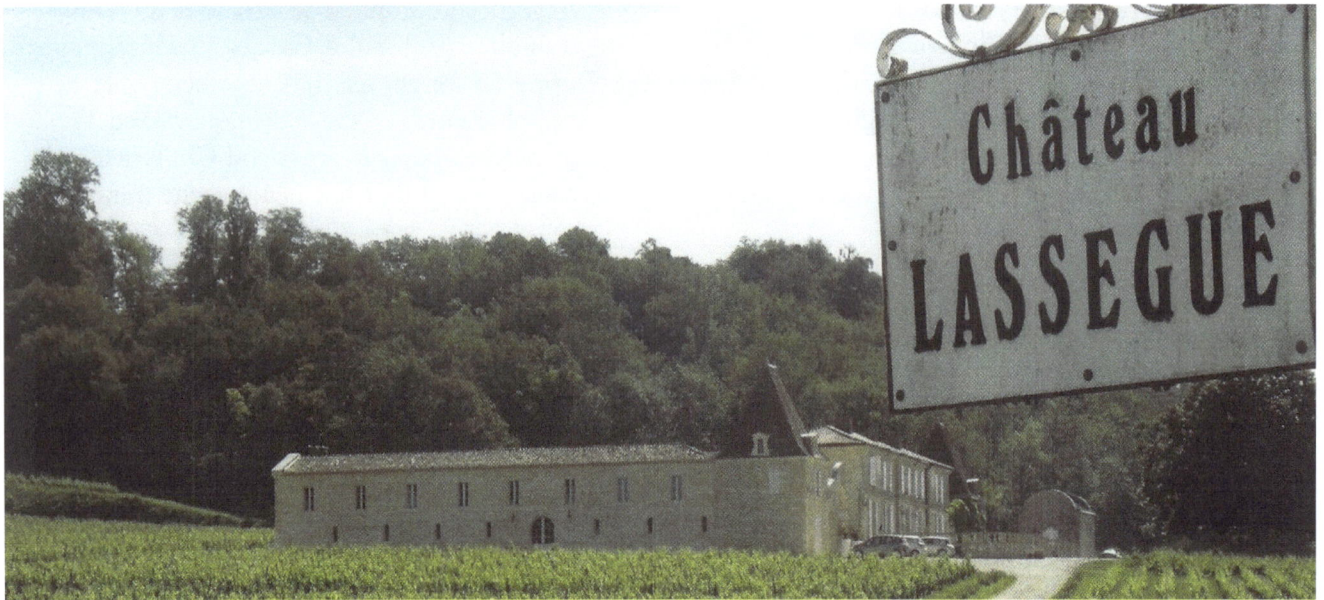

The southeast region is the oldest wine area of Bordeaux. Its wines are considered the most robust. They are generous, very colored, reaching their maturity quicker than other red Bordeaux. This vineyards did not grow in a day. The region has a rich, sometimes tumultuous history marked by Roman conquests in the 2nd. Century, barbarian invasions, English rule and many wars, finally leading to the great prosperity and reputation that Saint-Emilion enjoys today, been its basic varietals Merlot and Cabernet Franc grapes.

During the 8th century, a Benedictine monk named Emilion arrived on the "Pavie Plateau", and became known not only for his extreme kindness to others, but for the miracles he performed among the people of the region. He became a hermit, living in the limestone caves under the monolithic church, which he inspired. Once sainted, both the church and the town took on his name: Saint-Emilion. The king Louis XVI, centuries later, declared the high quality wines of Bordeaux's Saint Emilion to be the "Nectar des Dieux"or "Nectar of the Gods".

In December of 1999, the Saint-Emilion wine region was officially recognized as a "UNESCO World Heritage Site", a landscape of cultural significance. This glorifying citation acknowledges the exceptional universal acceptance, describing it as "a remarkable example of a historic winemaking landscape which has survived intact".

The winery of Chateau Lassegue is a living example of the Saint-Emilion excellency, nested in the beautiful 17th century Chateau. Natural virtues – perennial sun-drenched land, rich and diverse soils, exposure to coastal breezes – make up an estate as complex as the wines so skillfully produced from it by its proprietors, the Seillan and Jackson families. Chateau Lassegue combines the best of Old World

108

principles and New World techniques. Bathed in sunlight from dawn to dusk, the vineyards benefit from this saturation and by protection from chilly northern winds, a combination that encourages the best possible physiological maturity in the fruit. A nod to the land's sunny aspect, the Estate's frontage, is adorned with two vertical sundials (les cadrans in French), each vibrantly painted and equipped with a three-dimensional metal axial gnomon. More than 250 years old, the sundials were originally installed so vineyards laborers could track time while working. Still fully functional. The restored sundials serve as Chateau Lassegue's iconic emblem.

Let's elaborate on the jewels of the Chateau Lassegue. Saint Emilion Grand Cru collection's last outstanding releases:

The 2005 (60% Merlot – 35% Cabernet Franc – 5% Cabernet Sauvignon): This is considered as an EXTRAORDINARY vintage, one that you usually see only once in a lifetime. Vigneron Winemaster Pierre Seillan has said that "this has been the top of my career working in Bordeaux, after the 1982 vintage which was also an excellent year". Deep, dark red color. Very expressive bouquet of cashews, oregano, plums and cherry preserves. In the palate, charming strong aromatics with a superb acidity. Rich, intense and complex with very round tannins and a long finish.

The 2006 (55% Merlot – 37% Cabernet Franc – 8% Cabernet Sauvignon):This vintage is a different style than 2005, but within eight or ten years, there will be some nice surprises. With a beautiful ruby color, the wine has a beautiful fruit nose, clean and fresh. There are aromas of berry jam, a hint of roasted coffee and dark fruits, affirming a wine that tastes young. In the palate this wine is very harmonious with an elegant finish, light and fresh, despite the wine's power.

The 2007 (68% Merlot – 25% Cabernet Franc – 7% Cabernet Sauvignon): Produced from 40 to 50 years old vines. Presenting a deep garnet color, the wine has subtle aromas of leather with an expression of toasted bread and vanilla, developing into fresh black fruit and spices. It stays smooth and fresh until the end, with round and refined tannins. Extremely long and persistent finish.

Les Cadrans de Lassegue 2008 (60% Merlot – 25% Cabernet Franc – 15% Cabernet Sauvignon):
This second wine of Chateau Lassegue was born starting with this vintage. It has been named after the sundials (cadrans) which adorn the front of the Chateau, as symbols of the perfect sun exposure of the Estate. Wth an intense dark red color you can appreciate aromas of licorice, jammy dark fruits, plum, chocolate and vanilla. In the mouth, it evolves smoothly and expresses fine-grained tannins on the finish which will soften promptly.

Enjoy these wines kissed by the sun!

THE ORGANIC WINE

The oldest novelty in our Industry

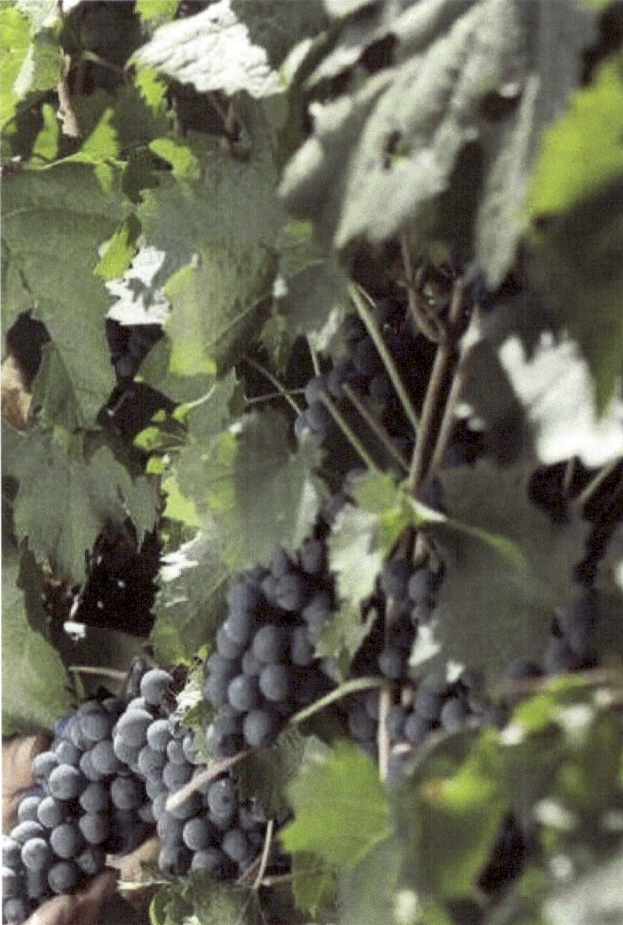

During the last decade the grape growers have opened the doors to the old style of the planting and raising of the grapevine, offering an alternative option for the lovers of wine. In the middle of the 1800s most of the European vineyards were destroyed by the effects of the *philoxera*, the most lethal and contagious biological plague that has been known in the history of the production of wine. The cure was not known; it cost millions and years of work of agricultural cleaning restoring the life of the grapevine territories. Since then, and to date, the intervention of Chemistry was instrumental in the prevention and finally in the eradication of the plague. This paved the way to the use of varied products manufactured by laboratories dedicated exclusively to this research, to achieve proper care and maximum development in the world of agriculture. Nevertheless, in this era, where one fights to renew and to improve our life style, the wine industry offers the option of returning to old times using the grapevine's organic cultivation, free of the influence of chemical agents. Certain confusion exists in "the organic" term.

The "100% organic wine" takes place with the traditional cultivation of the grape without the use of any synthetic fertilizers, pesticides, or bioengineering . Only the "sulfites" must be used in the process since it is the only way to fight the "oxidation" that shortens the life of the wine. All organic procedures must appear on the label and be certified by the corresponding institutions. Each one establishes the territorial parameters for nonorganic vineyards in order to avoid the chemical influence from the nonorganic *"terroirs"*. In the United States the USDA is the responsible government agency that insures compliance of this process.

From Argentina incomparable organic wines VINECOL, were produced since 1998.

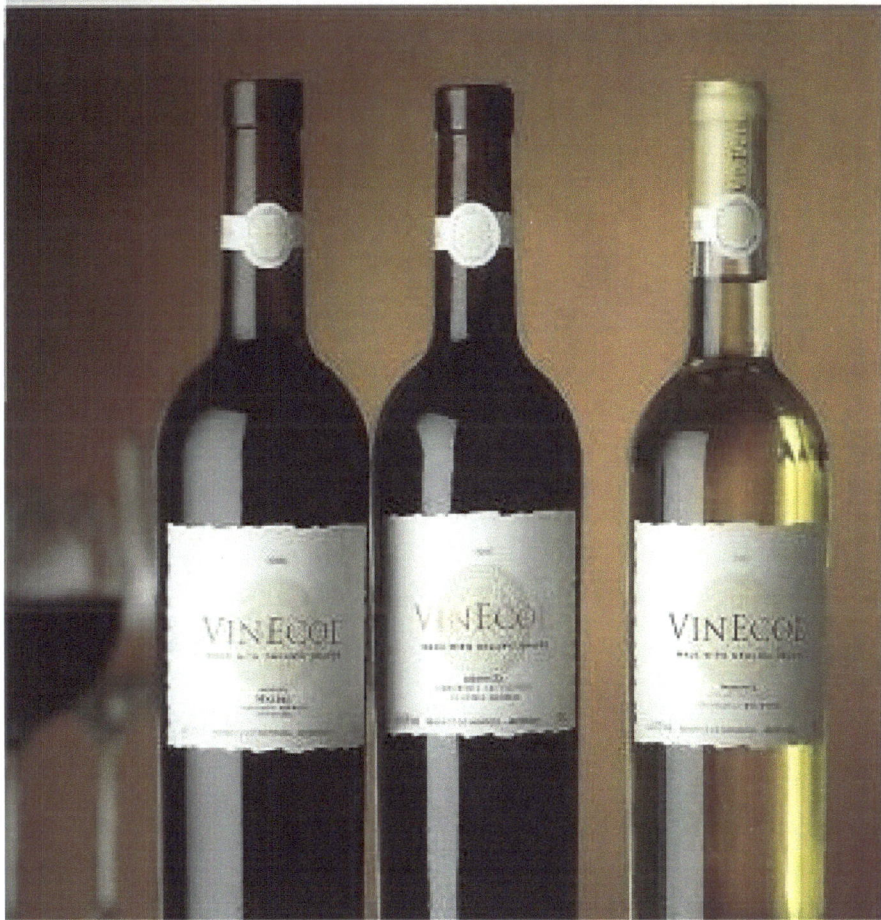

TORRONTES 2007: Pale gold color. A smooth wine filled with aromas of tropical fruits, fresh lemon and jazmin. Pleasent and persistent finale.

CHARDONNAY 2007: Brilliant gold color with emerald tones and aromas of creamy vanilla. In the palate vivid notes of creamy pears and apples, culminating in a prolonged finale.

MALBEC 2006: Red violet with ruby characteristics. Aromas of red plum, flowers and fruits. When tasting it an elegant and balanced structure is denoted with notes of French oak and flavor of spices.

CABERNET SAUVIGNON 2007: Brilliant ruby red color. Atarctive aromas of red fruits, black pepper and nuts. A long and spicy finale.

TEMPRANILLO 2007: Lively purplish red color. Complex and intense aromas of berries of the forest. In the palate creamy buttery notes and caramelized sugar is revealed. Persistent finale of strawberry flavor.

Now, when offering these wines, it is perfect to say "SALUD! "

THE BEAUJOLAIS WINES

George Duboeuf: illustrious representative of the most recognized wines of France

When referring about the wine industry, one can say that Beaujolais is "the third river" next to the Rhone and the Gaona that crosses the Languedoc and the city of Lyon, the second most populated in France.

This wine, the most recognized red wine in the world, has become through the centuries "an international sensation" due to its immense popularity and to the annual appearance in the market of its version Beaujolais Nouveau. By the strong character of its fruit and its casual style, this wine is also considered a symbol of hospitality, friendship, relaxation, commercial honesty and glamour without complications. Impossible to be reproduced in other regions, the variety of Gamay grape where these wines come from, is exclusively native to the Beaujolais soil. The George Duboeuf Bodega presents a unique display of wines, typically light, with radiant red cherry color and fruit of summer character, such as blacberry, currant and strawberry, defining its aroma and palate.

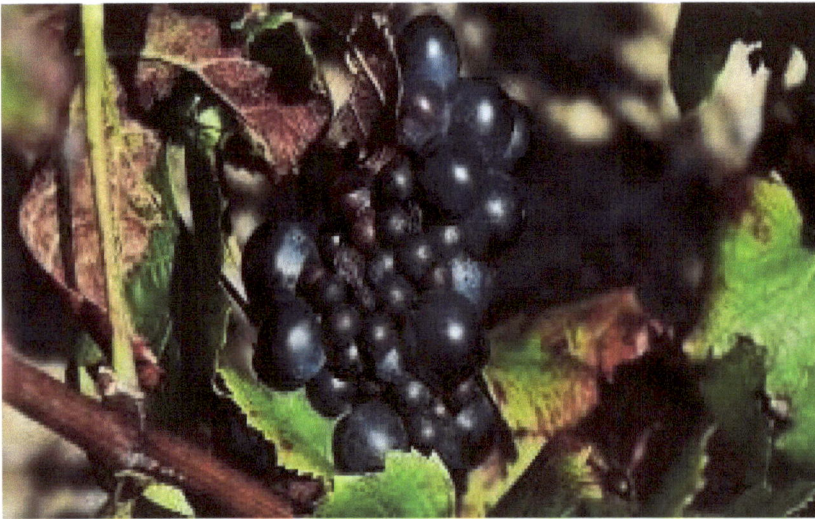

A short time back, George Duboeuf made a unique breakthrough of the typical French tradition by using smart blends for wine production. After a careful enological investigation of its vineyards, he selected certain areas to dedicate them to *varietal* wine production originated a 100% of a single species - a technique initiated in California during the 70s. – presented under the name Patch Block ("Isolated Land"), a selection of the most popular varietals in the wine world, offering consumers one of the most reasonable prices in the international market.

These are George's other marvels:

Sauvignon Blanc 2008: A sensually tempting golden white wine. Possesess strong fruit aromas, a shining flavor of tropical fruit with intense notes of fresh lime that lead to a round and long finale.

Chardonnay 2008: This golden beauty carries aromas of sweet almond, anise and citric fruits wrapped in a silky texture.

Cabernet Sauvignon 2008: A whole body wine with dark fruit and pepper aromas with a touch of mint. One denotes a lengthy and succulent chocolate-like finale.

Merlot 2008: Offers a strong black cherry aroma, giving the palate mocha-coffee and liquorice notes contributing to an intense finale.

Pinot Noir 2008: An exuberant wine with abundant currant flavors and mature cherries in a silky body with toasted and smoked notes.

Without failure, the launching of the Beaujolais Nouveau appears every year on November 21st.

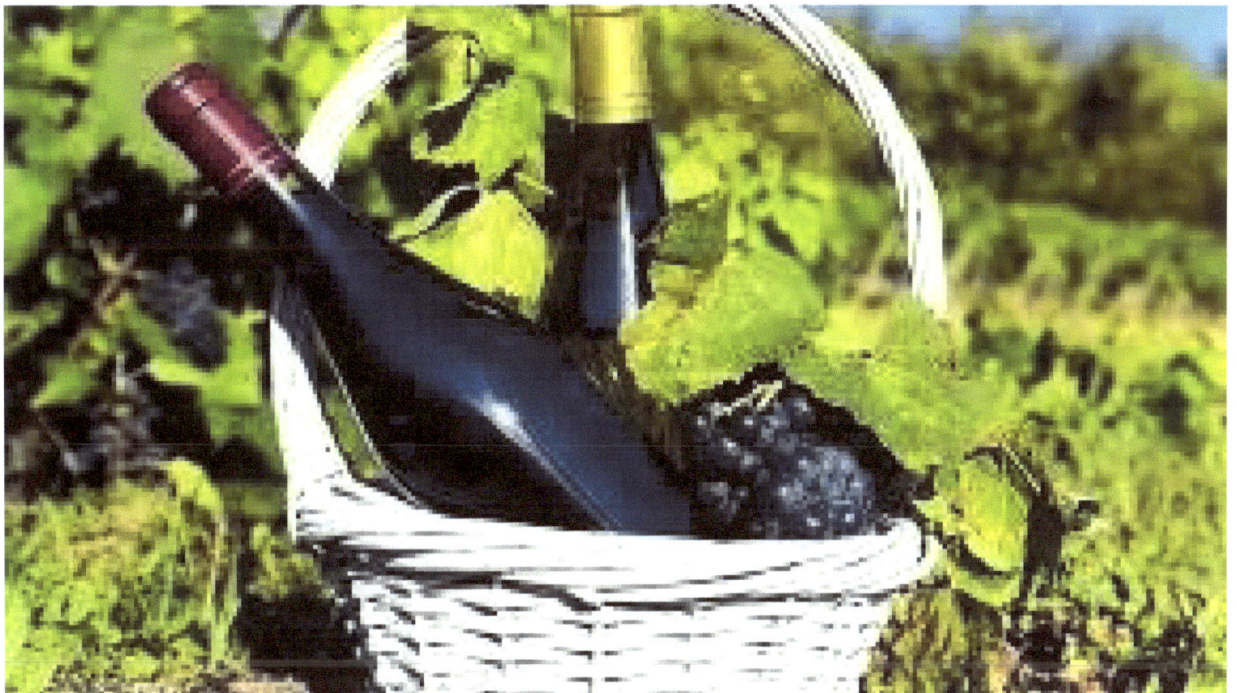

A LEGENDARY LINEAGE OF THE SCOTTISH CULTURE
The " Dalmore Single Malt", evoking an expression of a great Spírit

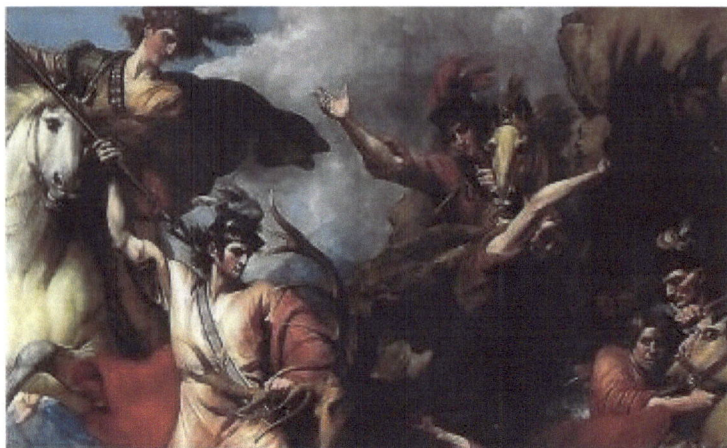

On April 15, 2005, someone paid 32,000 Sterling Pounds for one 65 year old bottle of Dalmore" Single Malt", containing an exceptional blend of illustrious whiskies pertaining to the 1868, 1878, 1922, 1926 and 1939. Only 12 bottles were produced. The buyer immediately ordered to open one of the bottles to experience, without delay, a masterpiece , giving the barman a tasting of the elixir as a tip. This legendary whisky was described by Jim Murray, author of *The Whisky Bible,* in the following terms: "Shining. Pure silk surrounding a a creamy fruit pie. Its aroma and flavor of the finest Oloroso Sherry defy nature by surviving in the barrel for such a long time. It leaves you dumbfounded. A unique whiskey in life".

The Dalmore distillery was founded in 1839 by Sir Alexander Matheson, businessman entrepeneur dedicated to the commerce of tea and tobacco from the Far East, which provided him with a great fortune. Later on he sold the distillery to the MacKenzie Clan, one of the most distinguished families in Scotland.

The Dalmore label was the result of an historical incident - dating from the year 1263 - in which a MacKenzie ancestor took part in a heroic Royal Hunting, lanceing a red deer that was on the verge of attacking King Alexander III. The Monarch, extremely grateful, proclaimed as standard of the Clan's Coat of Arms the image of a twelve horn stag. To date, it represents the commercial trademark of the more exclusive Single Malt in the industry.

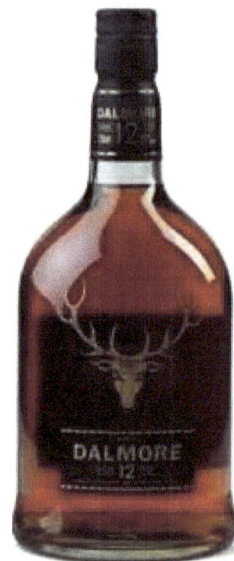

The distillery kept the gigantic copper stills originally installed in 1874. The Glasgow "Whyte and Mackay" current proprietors of "The Dalmore", acquired the company in 1960. Let's describe tthe Dalmore Collection:

THE 50: Time is the heart of this unique expression. Only 191 bottles were presented in artisan crystal and sent to the market, causing a great excitement among connoisseurs, gourmets and collectors throughout the world. A gold honey color, surrounds aromas of English style jam, ripe bananas, caramel and fruit pie. The palate shows Sherry, oak and orange notes. Cinnamon and almond finale. Cost $1,500.

114

***THE 40* (Double Gold Medal):** Barrelled in 1965, its bottling took years and many tastings. .Dressed in mahogany color, orange jam and Christmas pudding aromas are perceived. Bold caramel, bitter chocolate and almonds emits a lengthy finale. Cost $3,000.

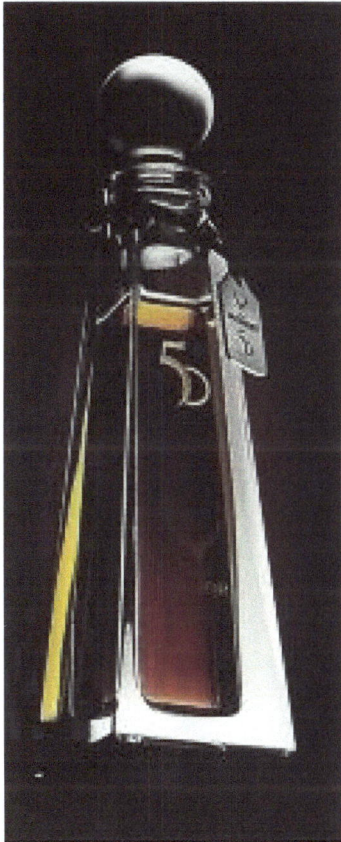

THE 1974 (Gold medal): The way to its perfection began in barrels used for "bourbon"distillation . 948 artistic bottles saw the light of day after being transferred to large "sherry" barrels for a second maturation, resulting in intense aromas of orange skin, cinnamon, chocolate and ripe bananas. Their flavors lock up notes of liquorice, apple compote, Java coffee and Sevillian oranges. Great nuts and dry fruit finale. Cost $1,250.

KING ALEXANDER III (Gold Medal): Barrels from different origins - Madeira, Port, Sherry, Sicilian Marsala and Kentucky Bourbon - were used to extract their spirit and transferred to this intense whiskey character. This wood macerating combination transfers to this variety a delightful vanilla flavor, crowned by notes of India berries of the forest and ripe plums.

THE 15 (Gold Medal): The perfect balance between spirit, wood and ripeness. Powerful, aromatic and robust. A whiskey with a heart filled with dry spices, cinnamon and ginger with a pleasant citric infusion.

THE GRAN RESERVA (Gold Medal): 10 to 15 years aged in White American oak (40%) and Oloroso Sherry (60%) barrels. Its elegant and refined body shows a touch of citric and autumn fruits and subtle roasted coffee and chocolate notes.

THE 12 (Gold Medal): This spirit balances the

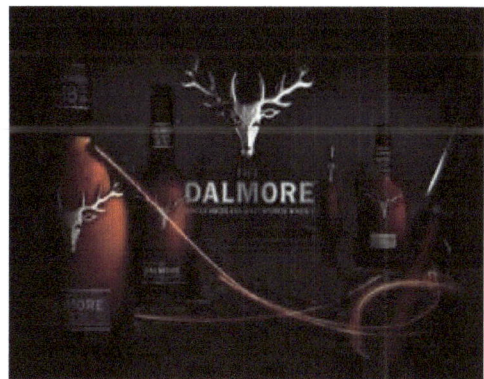

wood accurately, displaying both robustness and refinement at the same time, leaving a taste of shining complexity in the palate. With an intense mahogany color and interlaced jam, spicy aromas and a touch of vanilla, conducive to a lengthy finale.

"The Dalmore" is not simply a spirit, but a prestigious Single Malt collection of whiskeys, awarded with numerous medals in the San Francisco World Spirits Competition, opening wide the doors to the market in the United States.

A Single Malt worthy of admiration. Enjoy it!

THE WINES OF THE "TERRA D' ARGENTO"

The winery GRAFFIGNA ambassador of the highest excellence in winemaking

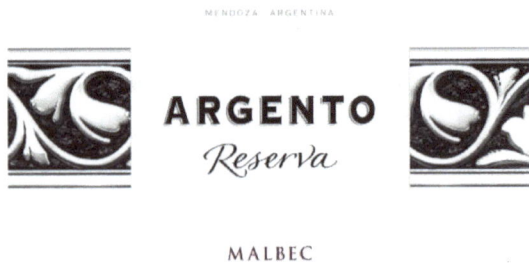

Argentina can be proud to have a wine culture monopolizing more than four hundred years of history. In the beginning of the XVI century, the Spanish settlers found in the slopes of the Andes a great variety of ideal microclimates for the "Vitis Vinifera" cultivation. The first record of existing vineyards goes back to the year 1557, in which, the Father Juan Citron, planted in the region of Santiago of the Matting, a version of the Mission grape variety from Spain. A wave of European immigrants, mainly proceding from Italy, Spain and France, settled down in the country from the beginning of the XVIII century, creating a profuse railway network interlacing Mendoza, the wine capital of the country with Patagonia, also reaching Buenos Aires. The settlers brought their wine production experience, and a great amount of European grapevines founding what is the greatest wine style diversity taking place in Argentina today.

A remarkable date in the country's winemaking trajectory was the appearance, in 1852, of the first planting of the Malbec variety, brought from France by the agronomist Michel Aimé Pouget. Presently, the Malbec is considered the official wine of Argentina, greatly recognized in the international market.

Don Juan Graffigna, a great italian expert in the Wine World, settled down in Argentina in 1865. At that time his wine business was first located in the region of San Juan. The transportation was inadequate, however, with the appearance of the railroad twenty years later, the Graffigna House, through generations, gradually became one of the most famous wineries in the country, offering optimal quality wines of great intrinsic value. After generations of arduous work, Graffigna is not only today the first "*bodega*" founded in San Juan, but it is also the second oldest in Argentina. Let us present the more recent jewels of the collection, 100% varietals, mainly coming from the *Valle del Pedernal* in San Juan. A great enological work:

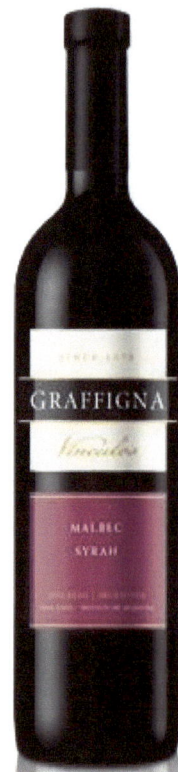

CENTENARY PINOT GRIGIO 2009: Coming from the Valley of Tulum (San Juan).

Color – Copperish green with golden notes.

Bouquet – White flowers aromas with a subtle peach touch.

Palate – Plenty of freshness and youth with smooth fruit notes and a pleasant finale .

Recommendations– Seafood in general, salmon and *"Risottos Fruta di Mare"*.

CENTENARIO MALBEC 2007: .
Color – Deep red with purple tones.
Bouquet – Aromas of dark fruits, black pepper and spices.
Palate – Complex flavor and balance, with mature tannins, vanilla and coffee notes.
Recommendations – Red meats, poultry, lamb and game.

GRAND RESERVE MALBEC 2007:
Color – Intense red-violet.
Bouquet – Red fruit, clove, cinnamon with smoky tones.
Palate - Mixture of new wood and tannins. Good structure and balance..
Recommendations – Perfect with red meat fillets and onion flavor in balsamic sauces

CENTENARIO CABERNET SAUVIGNON 2007:
Color - Intense ruby red with purple tones.
Bouquet – Red fruit aromas with tobacco and chocolate tones.
Palate – Affluent complex flavor with defined tannins and a vanilla touch.
Recommendations – Red meat skewers, stuffed baked chicken ,Curry sauces.

GRAND RESERVE CABERNET SAUVIGNON 2005:
Color – Deep ruby red.
Bouquet – Ripe fruit with flavors complemented with chocolate and tobacco notes.
Palate – Good structure and strong tannins with a touch of vanilla.
Recommendations – Grilled meats, fillet mignon, roasted pork.

To enjoy with "tango" and " tarantella". Salud!

THE DESSERT WINES
A good meal is incomplete without them

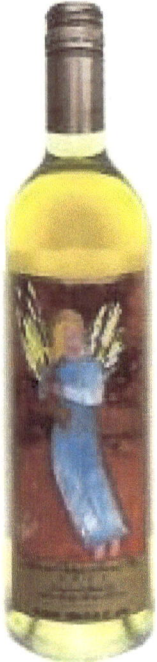

The sophisticated fashion to consume sweet wines accompanying exotic fruits and artisticly elaborated desserts, was introduced in the XVIII century in most European Royal Courts. As much as the gilded German Riesling and the French Sauternes of "noble rotting" or the fortified Tokay of Hungary, were imposed in the aristocracy's and rich bourgeoisie menus dominating the epicurean times of the "Good Table" that lasted until today. A magnificent dessert wine is not only a divine gift to the senses, but also the way to crown a glorious meal, followed by mixtures of distilled spirits, such special *"liqueurs"*. The wine industry has evolved progressively in the elaboration of sweet elixirs, conscious of its importance in a modern social diet. Certain countries, like Spain and Germany, produce diverse ideal varieties to accompany desserts, but is rare the wine region that does not cultivate some vineyards to elaborate this wine style.

In 1980, near Reedley, a town located south of Ash, in California, Andrew Quady, grape grower, enologist and founder of The Quady Winery, discovered a variety baptisted as "Orange Muscat", an almost unknown grape of Italian origin. As of that moment, with the unconditional help of his wife Laurel, Andrew Quady exclusively dedicated himsel in revealing to the consumer the high quality and exoticism of the California sweet wine. Let us elaborate on its creations:

ESSENSIA (100% Orange Muscat): The first wine sent to the market by the Quady Winery with 3 months of fermentation in barrels of French oak. Showing a Spanish Gold display and a vibrant orange spiced flavor. Magnificent with chocolate, it is also recommended with almond, peach, apple or apricot based desserts. Ideal for sprinkling sponge cakes and *"panetela"*. Mixed with soda water makes a refreshing "Spritzer" and with champagne offers s a sophisticated "Royal Essensia".

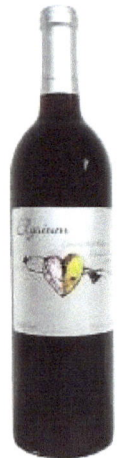

ELYSIUM (100% Muscat Hamburg): This Muscat grape is of black skin. The wine displays a crimson red color and develops aromas of lychee and roses. It is, without a doubt, great company for strong cheeses (gorgonzola, roquefort, blue cheese) and the best friend of desserts based in India berries, bitter chocolate or creamy combinations. Try it with vanilla ice cream an appetizing Elysium Sundae, also accompanied by a sip of Elysium.
.
ELECTRA (100% Orange Muscat): Similar to Essensia but of low alcoholic content. Magnificent with fresh fruits (strawberries, tangerins, peaches and melon) and a great companion of salads and Oriental dishes. Electra is a pic-nic wine for warm climates. (4% Alcohol). A second version is "Electra Red".

DEVIATION (100% Orange Muscat and herbal infusion): Its name reveals a "diverted" wine process. It is produced by mixing aromatic herbs, "Pelargonium" (pink geranium) native of South Africa and "Damiana" from Mexican and South America tropical areas combined with the Orange Muscat grapes. The result is an exciting and uniquely flavored dessert wine. Excellent as a digestive.

BATCH 88 STARBOARD & QUADY'S STARBOARD 1996: Even though this is an "*Oporto*" or PortWine, Andrew Quady decided to name it "Starboard" since the climate and the soil of his California property   is significantely different from Portugal. The grape varieties used are "Tinta Roriz", "Touriga Nacional" y "Tinta Cao" were imported from the *Duero* River Valley, cradle of the Portuguese Oporto, allowing the production of a delicious wine with big body and character, of a silky raisin and chocolate flavor.

We must leave the best for last !

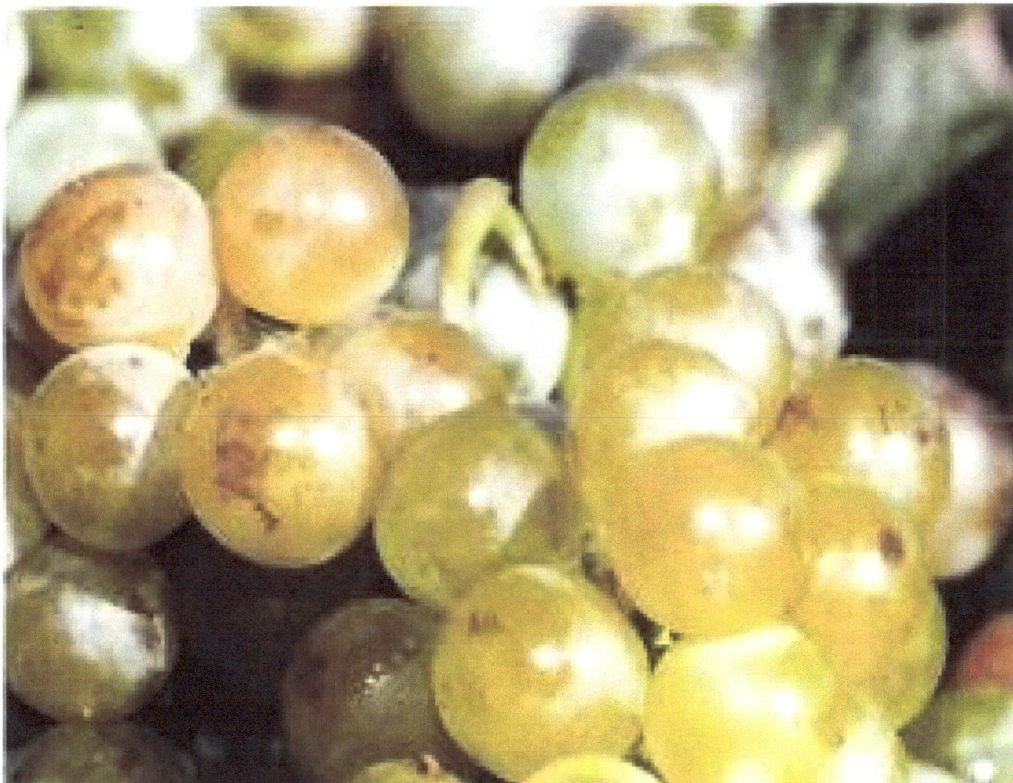

LOUIS XIII

Debut of "Le Jeroboam", the greatest Cognac of the Rémy Martin House

Considered the most complex and esteemed spirit of the world, the Cognac Louis XIII, pinnacle of the creations of the Rémy Martin House, is a unique *"acqua vitae"* combination of multiple "wáter of life" coming from the finest vineyards Grande Champagne of the Cognac region. Celebrating the historical legacy of excellence that Emile Rémy Martin initiated with his introduction many years back. A new Louis XIII version majestically made its appearance in a Jeroboam, artisan three liters Baccarat crystal bottle.

The incredible history of Louis XIII begins in 1874, thanks to the shining vision of Paul Emile Rémy Martin. He made a mixture of the most aged "waters of life" of its *"bodega"* and bottled it in an exact metal "decanter" replica adorned with *Fleurs de Lis* lost during the XVI century in the battlefield of Jarnac, found 300 years later.

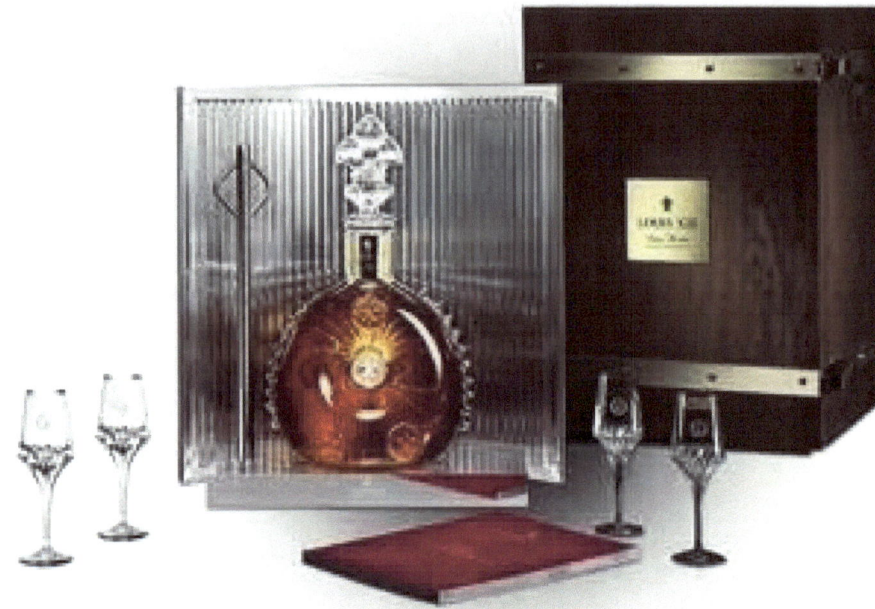

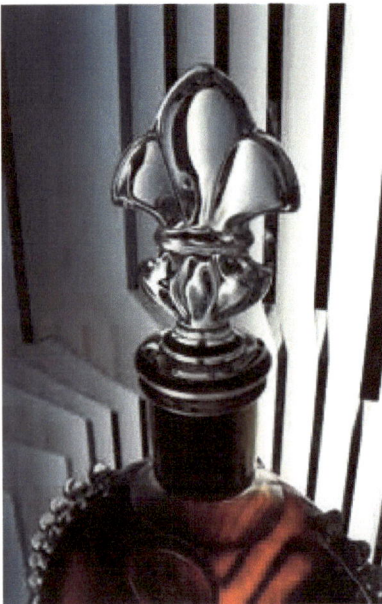

This magic elixir is result of the blend of 1.200 "waters of life" aged for more than one hundred years, all exclusively coming from the most reputable vineyards of the Cognac región.

.

Louis XIII is the oldest and finest of cognacs, product of a magical combination of *"savoir faire"*, art, patience and expert knowledge of the spirits world.

Four generations of Master Distillers have supervised the production of the elixir for more than a hundred years, watching the aging methods and blend control that result in great harmony, matchless elegance and *bouquet* generosity. "To obtain happiness is a team effort" commented Pierrette Trichet, presently Remy Martin House Master Distiller:
"I am only a link in the chain. Great cognacs are developed through the passage of several professional generations".

Considered around the globe by its rich legacy of innovation and superior merit, combined with intense and complex aromas of iconic spirit, Louis XIII has always been considered a symbol of prestige, taking part in many of the most famous events in history. Some examples includes the first intriguing and romantic travels in the *"Orient Express"* (1929); the first transoceanic trip of *"Le Normandie"* to New York (1935) and the first supersonic flight aboard the *"Concorde"* (1984). Served in most of the European Royal Courts, *Louis XIII* adorns t h e R o y a l T a b l e s as an *"art de vivre"* Ambassador.

Shortly, his *Jeroboam* is an investment for the consumer of luxury, with the taste by the finest Cognac or for the collectors of objects of the most appreciated value. Cost: $26,000.

A unique experience

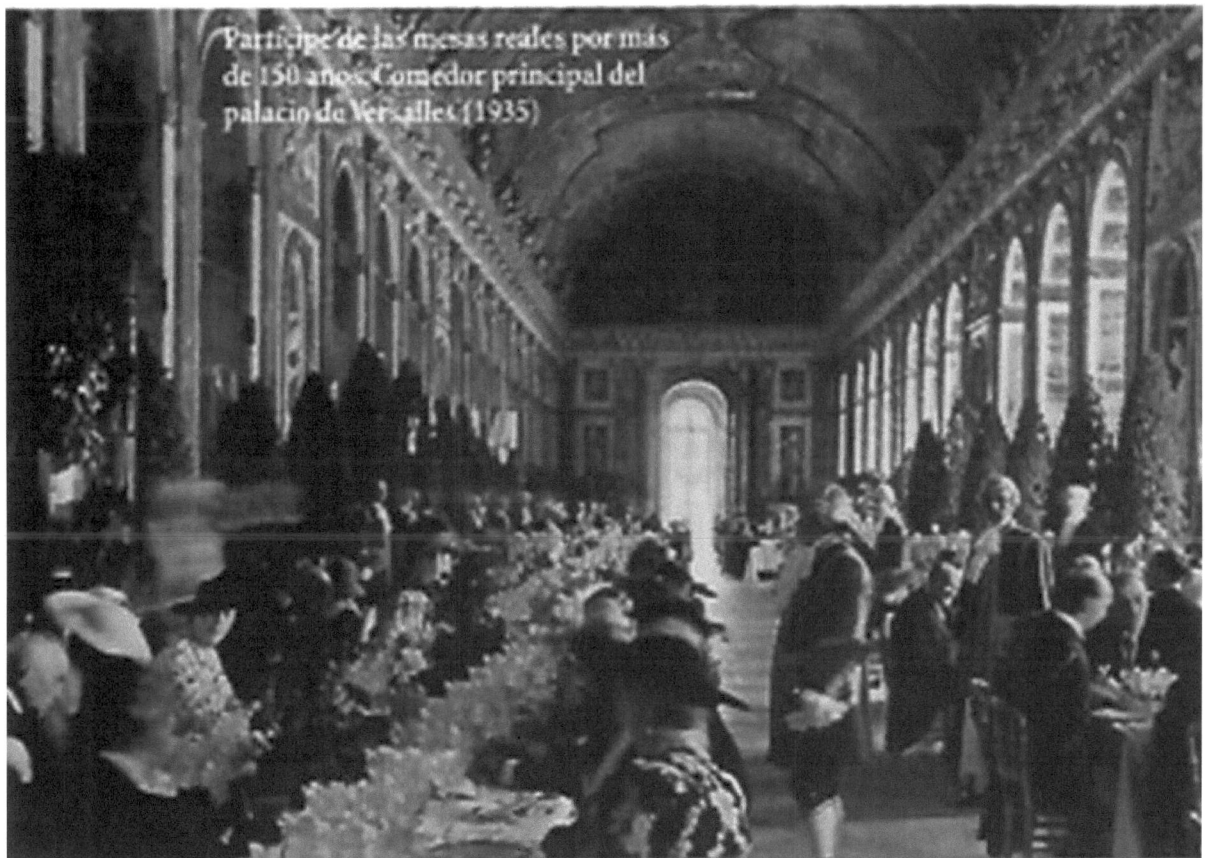

Participe de las mesas reales por más de 150 años. Comedor principal del palacio de Versalles (1935)

INDOMITABLE TENACITY AND GLORIOUS EXCELLENCE

The BACARDI HOUSE celebrates its 150 anniversary presenting its Commemorative Bottle

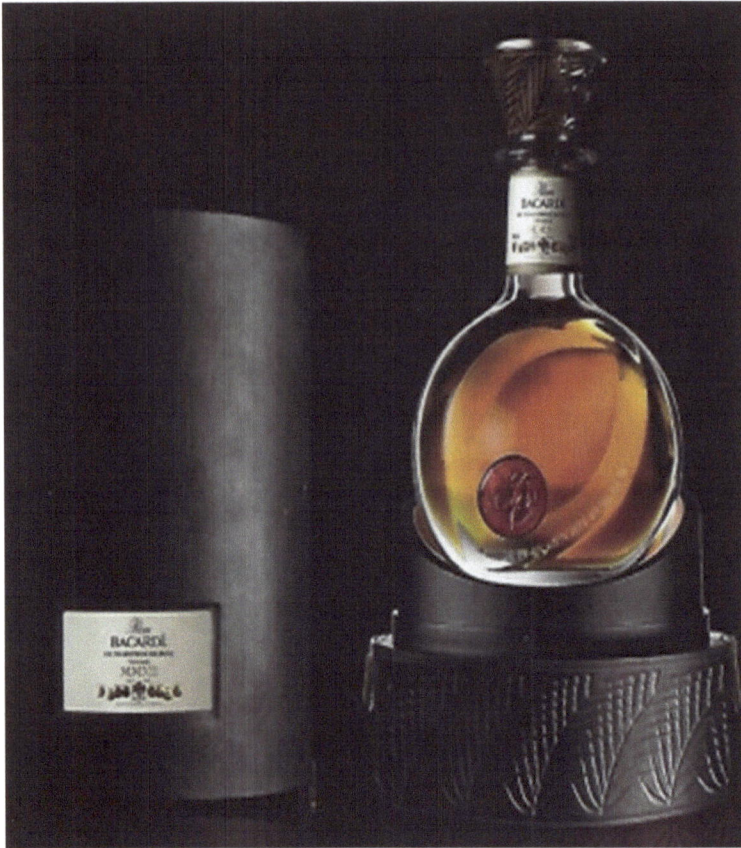

BACARDI was created in *Santiago de Cuba* the 4 of February of 1862, when Don Facundo Bacardi Massó bought a small distillery.

After years of experimentation, Bacardi revolutionized the industry of the spirits when adding steps that never had been used in the elaboration of rum. It selected residual sugar cane molasses of high quality, isolated a special leavening stock - that still is used today, - it filtered and it matured his rums in North American white oak barrels, and later mixed them to obtain the "perfect flavor".

The smooth and slight drink that was created, in opposition to the rough brandy of then, was BACARDI - the first rum of high class of the world and the first rum that can be combined, giving origin to the culture of the "cocktail" that dominates the social scope of today. The ingenious Teachers of Rum follow the same demanding norms settled down by Don Facundo.

"During the last 150 years, Bacardi, like family, a company and a mark - has reunited to people in legendary celebrations and delicious cocktails. Visit any bar, club or restaurant almost anywhere in the world, and the impact that Bacardi has caused in the industry of the spirits is clearly visible", affirms Seamus McBride, President and Executive Director (CEO) of Bacardi Limited.

"It is incredible to see a company of a single Brand, established for 150 years, has become the third power of spirits in the world, with an enviable portfolio of iconic liquors that includes the vodka GREY GOOSE, the gin BOMBAY SAPPHIRE, Scottish whiskey DEWAR' S, vermouth MARTINI, vodka ERISTOFF and HUNTING tequila 100% of blue "*agave*".

Celebrations for the anniversary of BACARDI have taken place almost everywhere in the world, presenting awarded artistic and musical talents, celebrities and many other influencial people, next to the consumers, wishing BACARDI a Happy 150th Birthday.

Germany initially opened the celebrations, next to Canada and the United States. Most of Europe, Latin America, Pacific Asia and the Middle East were also united in the tribute. The guests celebrated with legendary RUM BACARDI cocktails, some created more than a 100 years ago, including the most popular of the world, the originals "Cuba Libre", "Daikiri", "Mojito" and "Piña Colada".

Since the RUM BACARDI *debut* in the market, the consumers have enjoyed more than 365 million of cocktails. That means that every second of the day more than 200 BACARDI cocktails are tasted anywhere in the world.

To commemorate this Anniversary, BACARDI has created a Baccarat crystal decanter with a genuine leather cover, that contains an aged combination of rums matured for 20 years in Cognac barrels of 60 years of life. Cost US $2,000.

"The passion and the enterprising spirit that my Great Great Grandfather showed in *Santiago de Cuba* 150 years ago, created an exceptional Rum industry forever." Words of Facundo L. Bacardí (Fifth generation of the family).

Let's make a toast to this Anniversary!

THE VIBRANT RIOJA

Spain introduces its tradition and "new wave" Wines

Miami was the host of a great enological event, "The Vibrant Rioja", about the international caliber of the Spanish wine. New York, Chicago and San Francisco preceeded the City of Sun in the celebration of this "IV Great Tasting". La Rioja is technically the oldest wine region in Spain, presentsing us with a constant evolution, combining a perfect balance between tradition and innovation. This event, was about the great mutual compatibility between the excellence and quality of its wines, conducted by a new generation of proprietors of great enological talent. The attendants had the opportunity to taste more than 200 Riojas, mainly red, represented by 50 wine import companies. Presenting:

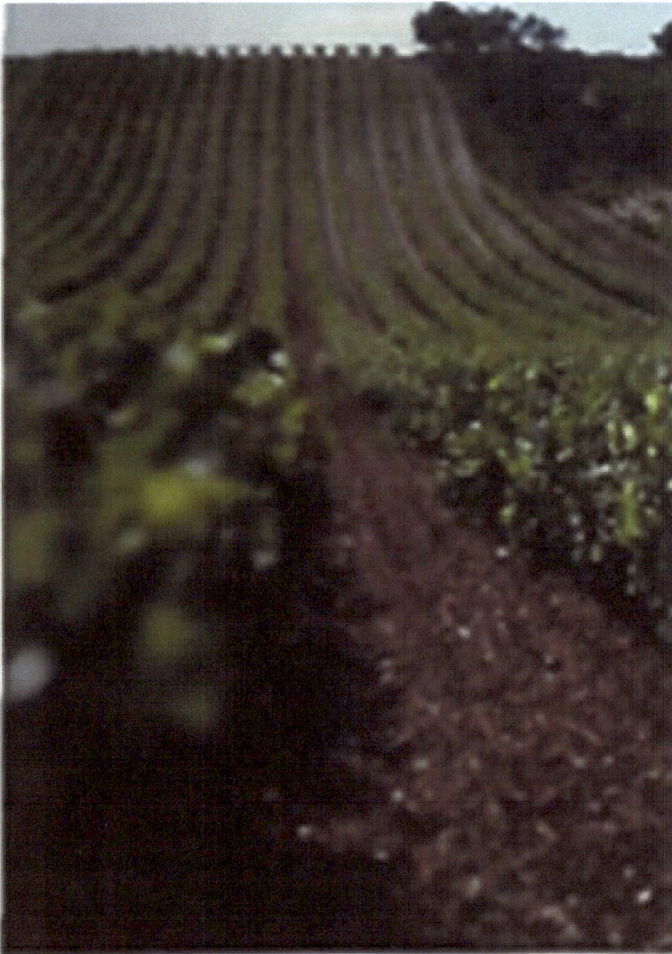

"Castillo de Ygay 2004". Great Special Reserve (93% Tempranillo - 7% Mazuelo): An elegant classic wine of deep red garnet color, with dark fruit aromas and a great body. Castilo de Ygay, from the "Marqués de Murrieta" winery is exclusively bottled in the best harvest years. Ideal to accompany roasted red meats, game, cured ham and strong cheeses.

"Conde de Valdemar 2005". Reserve (90% Tempranillo - 10% Mazuelo): Of a shining red cherry color, with vanilla, cedar and spice aromas. This great Reserve is perfectly balanced by its excellent acidity and medium tannins conducting us to a smooth and long finale. A great companion of roasted meats, grilled hunt and semismooth cheeses.

"Barón de Ley 7 Viñas 2005" (55% Tempranillo – 15% Garnacha – 15% Graciano – 7% Viura – 5% Malvasia and 2% White Garnacha): An impressive replica of "Viejo Rioja". As a tribute to the traditional style of winemaking, Baron de Ley 7 Viñas contains, in different percentages, the spirit of the seven grape varieties allowed by the Denomination of Origin regulations in La Rioja. The color is mulberry deep of shining edge. Aromas of ripe India berries combined with floral violet fragrances. In the palate, presents a perfectly balanced, elegant wine of smooth tannins. To serve it with appetizer, poultry, meats in general and all cheeses.

"Ontañón 2004". Reserva (85% Tempranillo – 15% Graciano): The grapes used for the production of this wine come from the most beautiful old stocks and rare family vineyards. A classic red with a naturally balanced acidity, result of its cultivation at more than 700 meters of altitude. It emanates intense aromas of ripe fruit with mineral outlines and dark chocolate. This wine is only produced in years of exceptional harvest. It is recommended with red meats, cured cheeses and *patés*.

Salud! Savouring the newest Spanish Rioja wines

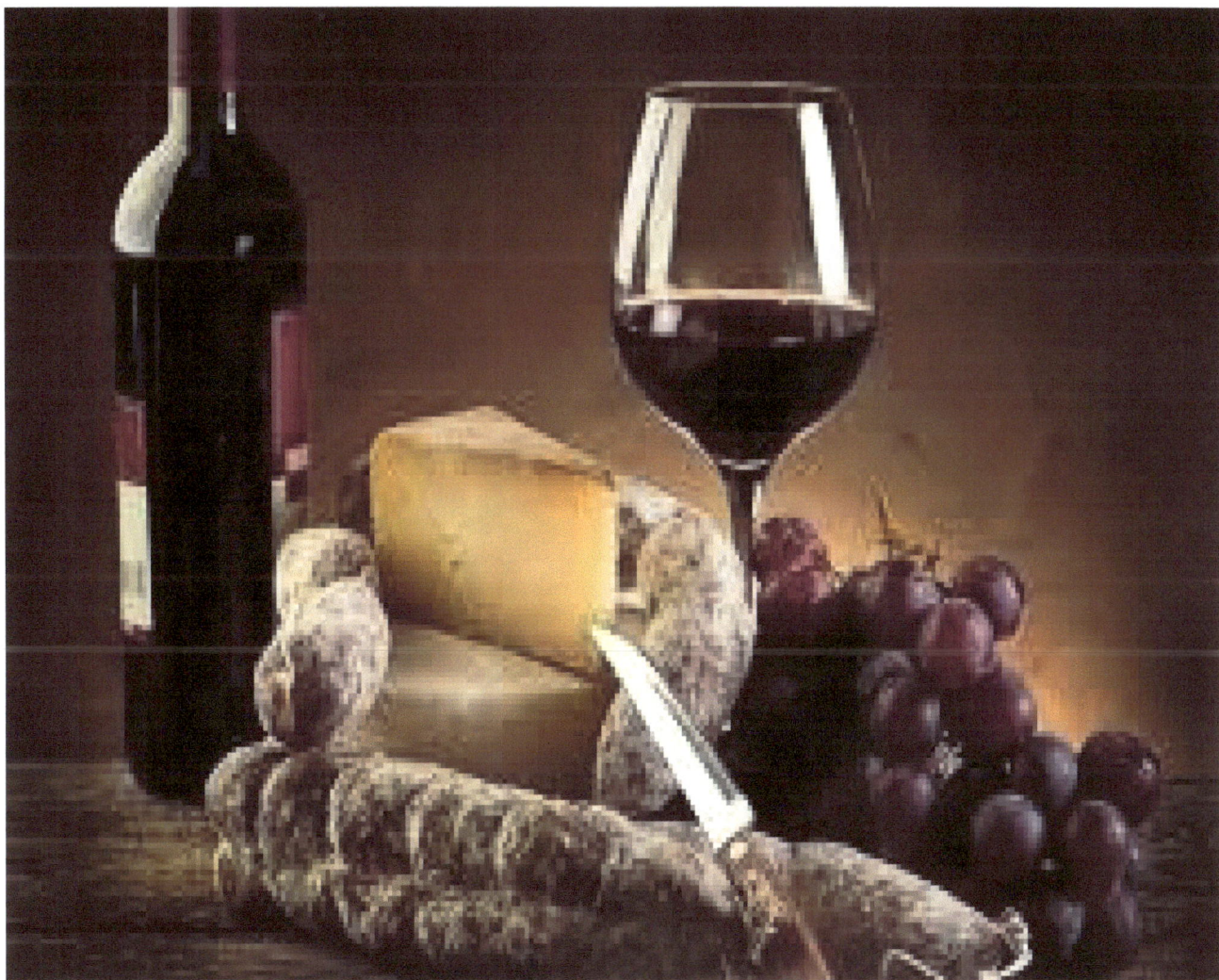

THE UNIVERSALLY POPULAR PINOT GRIGIO
A Glory of Italy

Few white wines have reached the peak of the Market in such a brief time as the PINOT GRIGIO. It was the Italian Master Enologists, the ones that adquired with this wine a spectacular reputation among the wine lovers, particularly in the United States, where it enjoys a great popularity. It is smooth and refreshing being the first option in celebrations of all types, visits to restaurants and domestic consumption.

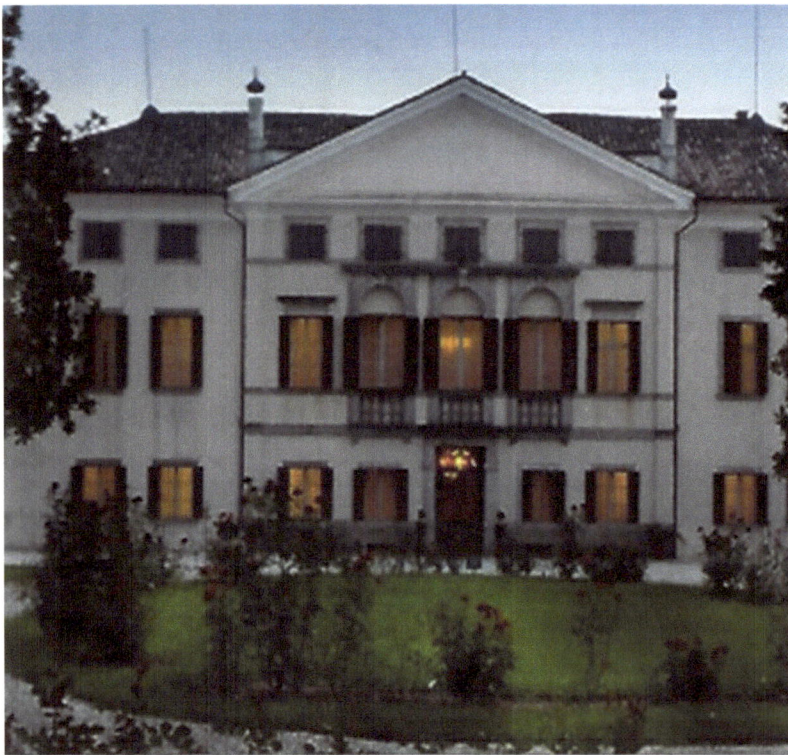

Pinot Grigio is originally a derivative of the Pinot Gris french variety, which never had much success in the international market, opposite to the Pinot Grigio which is recognized as a masterpiece in Europe and the Americas. Italy, being this elixir's "mom" is its great producer, due to its terroir of optimal weather conditions. The Bodegas Pighin & Figli, are the architects of a Pinot Grigio of great quality and high tradition, owned by this aristocratic Italian family since 1963.

Located in Friuli, PIGHIN is technically considered the more outpost wine producer. We also must mention their Sauvignon Blanc, also a result of its enological wisdom. Presenting the jewels of the collection:

PINOT GRIGIO FRIULI GRAVE 2010 (100% Pinot Grigio) : A wine of a shining gold color and an amber shade. With a medium body texture, shows candied aromas of banana and pear in its bouquet and palate, with a caressing acidity. Developes well in the bottle by up to four years. Alcohol: 12.4%

Recommendations: Magnificent with poultry, fresh fish and seafood, light pasta dishes, vegetarian creations and smooth cheeses.

PINOT GRIGIO COLLIO 2009 (100% Pinot Grigio): Of a pale yellow color emanates atractive citric notes. It confers a fresh acidity to the palate, presenting a surprising body and great mineral personality with notes of pear and apple. Clean and fresh finale. Alcohol: 13%
Recommendations: Ideal with white fish and seafood, sushi, vegetable risotto, poultry and veal dishes.
.
SAUVIGNON FRIULI GRAVE 2011 (100% Sauvignon Blanc): Pale yellow color. The wine shows persistent tomato leaves aromas, with notes of green pepper and wild flowers. Is an elegant wine in the palate displaying fresh and intense flavors conducting us to an excellent and long finale.
Alcohol: 12.5%. Recomendations: Creamy vegetable soups, soufflés, and also great with salami.

The wine for all pleasures!

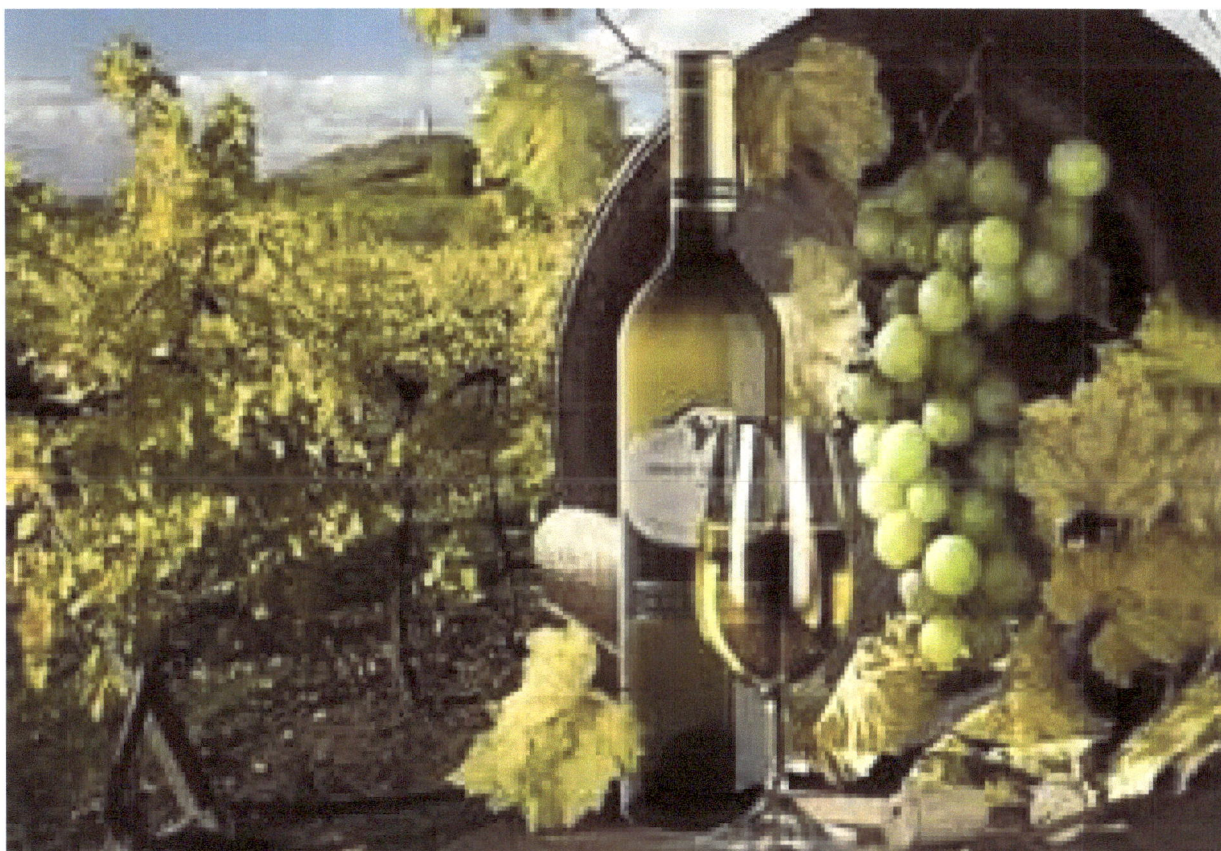

THE CARRIER OF THE SCOTTISH WHISKEY BANNER

"The Macallan" Single Malt presents its new and exclusive collection.

After 1814, the travellers in Scotland had to cross the famous bridge on the Spey river where surged "The Macallan". Its name was created of the combination of two words coming from the Gaelic language, "MAGH", meaning "Fertile Earth" and "ELLAN", referring to "San Fillan", the Irish monk who tirelessly preached Christianity in Scotland. In centuries, its inhabitants distilled whiskey of barley grain cultivated in their own soils.

The new millenium has been a witness of "Macallan" greatest success. In 2004 received its sixth *"Queen' s Award for Enterprise"*, proclaimed by its excellence, also receiving *"Single Malt No 1 of Scotland"*, distilled exclusively from barley Malt. In 2005, a bottle of *"The Macallan Fine and Rare Collection 1926"* won a *"Sterling Price"* of 36.000 Pounds, the largest amount paid in auction. That same year *"The Macallan Fine Oak"* appeared in the market receiving a world-wide aclamation. Later on, in 2006, emerged the *"Macallan & Lalique"* long aged whiskeys bottled in exclusive crystal cut bottles, the classiest in the world. This jewell collection of spirits consists in:

Macallan& Lalique 50 Years Old, $5,995.00.
COLOR: Midnight Sun and Old Gold.
AROMA: Notes of spices and intense *marraschino* notes.
PALATE: Aromatic dark plums and chocolate.

55 Years Old, $14,000.
COLOR: Dark Palisandro Tree.
AROMA: Sweet and exotic dry fruits with a smoked touch.
PALATE: Smooth and silky with citrus and of spicy notes.

57 Years Old, $15,000.
COLOR: Intense mahogany.
AROMA: Ginger, raisins and orange and notes of oak and vainilla.

60 Years Old, $20,000.
COLOR: Deep copper.
AROMA: Complex notes of cinnamon, toasted apple and lemon, combined with blackberry leafs.
PALATE: Sweet citrus and smoked dark chocolate. The distillery, built in 1700, is a great pride sample by its *"Six Pillars of Macallan"*: this classic property faces the fields, hills and rivers of Scotland, displaying:
Peculiarly small stills: These are a unique size stills to assure a maximum contact with copper, helping the elixir concentration.

Exceptional oak barrels: Handmade, chosen of from the vast distellery. The finest cut: Only 16% of the distills are selected to take place in the maturing barrels, being a robust symbol of the "new style" beginning of "Macallan".´

Natural color: The fact of choosing the most exceptional barrels gives the spirit a wonderful variety of crystalline colors. Selective moment: To watch constantly if, at any moment, each barrel is in its top maturity and the spirit is in perfect shape. This masterful combination is the secret of the creation of the "better whiskey of the world".

The complete line "The Macallan" presents today the following variety: 10 Yrs. - 12 Yrs. - 15 Yrs. - 17 Yrs. - 18 Yrs. - 21 Yrs and 25 Yrs.

To accompany with Bagpipe musique!

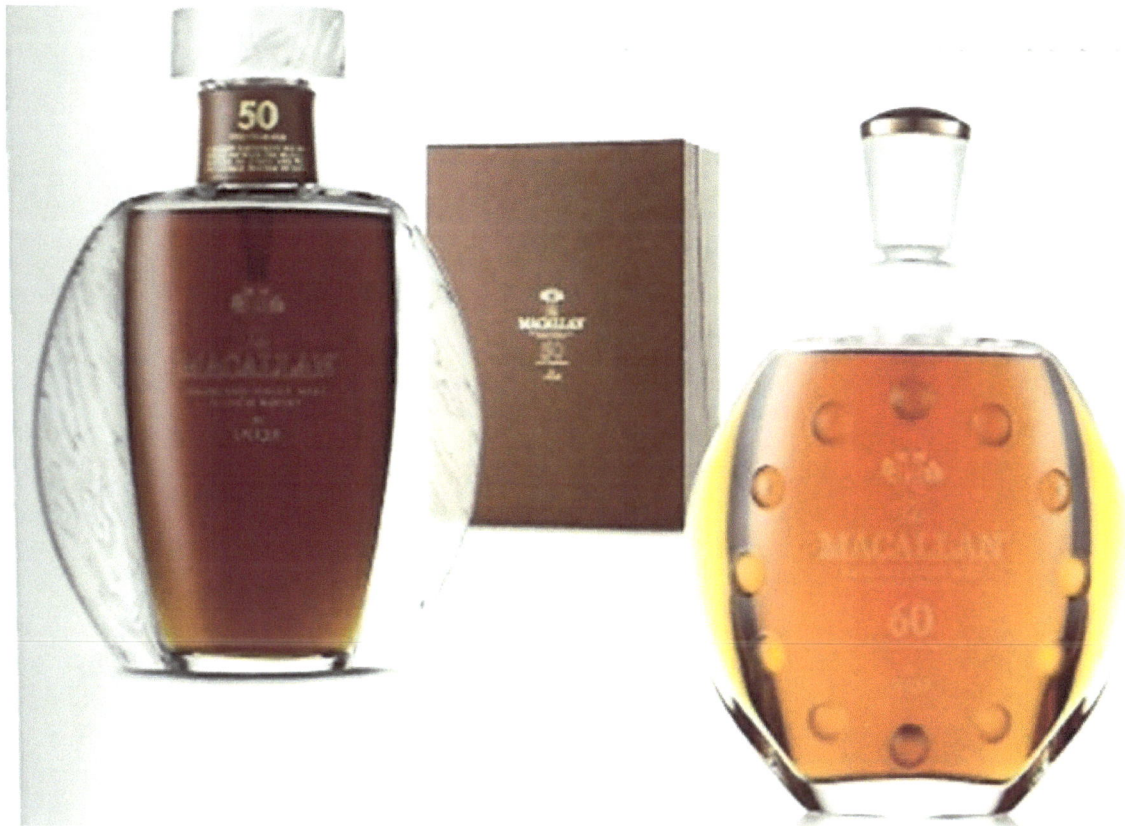

MY MORE PRECIOUS WINES ARE WATCHED BY SATAN HIMSELF
Warning in the *"Concha y Toro"* winery

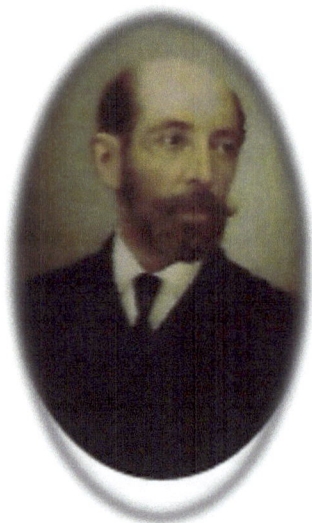

In the last years of the XIX century, *Don Melchor de Concha y Toro*, an eminent Chilean Man of State, brilliant trader and owner of vineyards, discovered that his more appreciated wines had been removed from the winery's private cellars of his ancestral house. In order to prevent these robberies, he spread the rumor that its deep and dark *Bodega* were enchanted by the Devil, eternal watchman of his jewels in *"casilleros"*. Then the legend was born of "Devil's Square", keeping safe the wines, nowadays, best sold around the world. The original winery, *"Hacienda Concha y Toro"*, with its picturesque "Square", is today the greater tourist attraction in Chile.

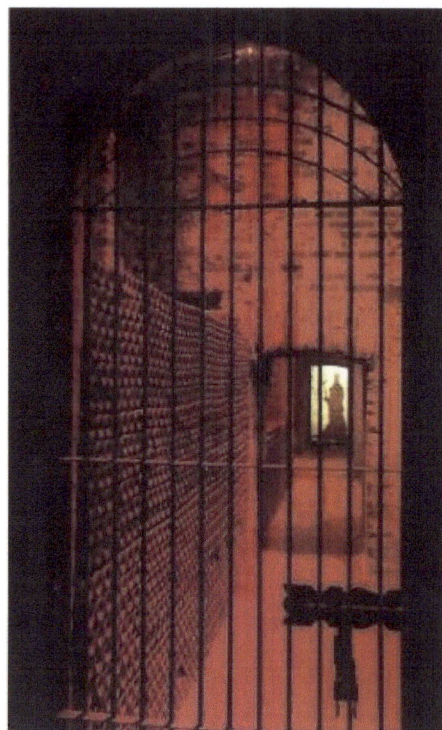

Perhaps the wines are stored hypothetically in hell, but they are the product of an authentic enological paradise. With sun light, enjoyment, fresh winds, vines inmune to phylloxera, great *terroir* extensions and experienced workers, Chile is the dream of a wine producer. Adding its long tradition based in the use of the most renowned varieties of French grapes and advanced production techniques, we have a Grand Prize combination. Thanks to its highest wine quality and great intrinsic value the company became one of the first producers in exporting wine to the United States. Let's elaborate:

"CASILLERO DEL DIABLO" (100% Cabernet Sauvignon) In 1953 made its launching in the market, being introduced in the United States in 1966. Since 1998, Prizes and Honorary Mentions fluorish for the company, reaching the zenith of the Industry, invigorating the"*Devil's Square"* and winning **The Wine Cellar of the Year award**.

The "Devil's Square" line of wines is extensive, consisting mainly of the following creations: CABERNET SAUVIGNON, CARMÈNERE, MERLOT, PINOT NOIR, MALBEC, WINEMAKER' S PRIVATE RESERVE NETWORK, CABERNET, SAUVIGNON, SYRAH RESERVE, MALBEC PRIVATE LABEL, CHARDONNAY and SAUVIGNON BLANC. Let's describe the best wines from this numerous collection:

CABERNET SAUVIGNON: (100%Cabernet Sauvignon): This classic is the standard wine of "Devil's Square". Presents an intense red ruby color, with aromas of cherries, raisins and black plums. High concentration, rich in flavor, perfectly balanced with a persistent finale. Because of its great structure is recommended with roasts, stews, game and all cheeses.

130

CARMENÈRE (100% Carmenère): This variety is considered the official grape of Chile. It shows a deep violet color, carrying aromas of black plums and chocolate with a touch of coffee and toast. It shows a great body and structure, framed by toasted American oak. Great with red meats, smooth pasta dishes and all cheeses.

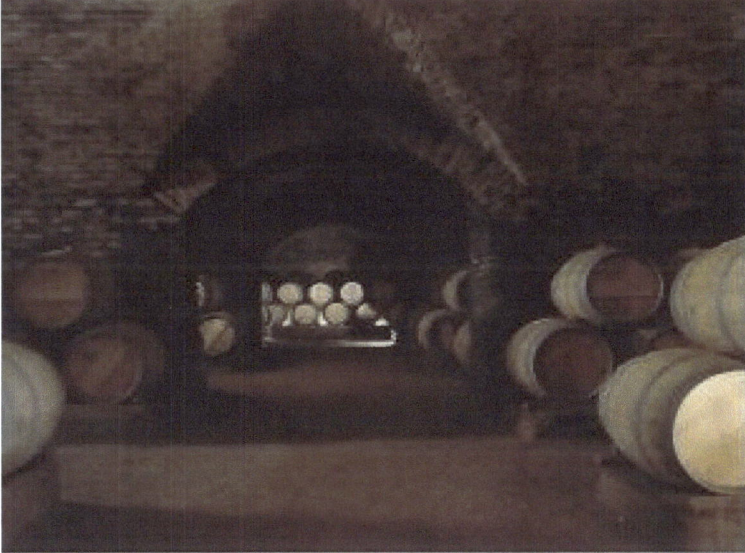

MALBEC (100% Malbec): With a purple violette color, presents aromas of dark fruit with a touch of spice. Flavors of plums, spices and cocoa, caresses the palate with a long finale. Magnificent with barbecues and vegetables. Great firm cheeses companion.

PINOT NOIR (100% Pinot Noir) Presents a shining raspberry red color. Aromas of bilberries are raisins and pomegranate are detected and balanced with a good acidity. A wine of medium viscosity showing a finale with a touch of spices. Recommended with white meats, poultry and fresh fruit salads.

CHARDONNAY (100% Chardonnay): An expressive and elegant wine. Shining an attractive lemon-yellow color, presents aromas of pomgranate and citric fruits. A perfectly balanced wine, with a shining acidity and a memorable long finale. Great to accompany seafood, poultry, pastas with light sauces and most cheeses.

SAUVIGNON BLANC (100% Sauvignon Blanc): Straw color with greenish tones. A wine of fresh and attractive aromas displaying a touch of citrus, peach and wild currant. A round wine of crushing acidity that transports you to a long and festive finale. Fastantic companion of fresh fish and seafood such as clams and oysters.

If Lucifer had tasted them, these wines would be all gone!

FROM THE "RIA BAIXAS" OF GALICIA
"Albariño Martin Códax" its distinguish Ambassador

In 1986 the Winery Martin Códax is born taking the name of one of the most famous Galician trovator with his Galaico-Portuguese *"cantigas"*, singing to "Love" and the *"Rias Baixas"* by the Cantabrian Sea, prevailing to date in the Galaico-Portuguese Folklore. From the beginning, the Winery has evolved always supporting the ancient culture of its people.

This project began with the illusion and the effort of a large group of grape growers. Nowadays it is already a reality that has turned the Martin Códax Winery into a Galician wine emblem. Their elixirs are produced following modern techniques without forgetting the traditional methods.

Its vineyards, divided in small parcels, are characterized for the classic system of vine cultivation and taken with great care by a highly technical personnel of grape growers for obtaining the maximum possible quality. The harvest begins in the middle of September, mainly manually, and the clusters carefully deposited in boxes of no more than 20 kg. in order to avoid squashing preserving its quality. Once in the Winery and analized for a full cleaning, the grapes are deposited in a pneumatic press to extract the juice or "mosto". Right after, begins the alcoholic fermentation process carried out in 30,000 stainless steel tanks. Once finished, begins the malolactic fermentation, that transforms the malic acids into lactic, thereby avoiding excessive acidity. Finally, the wine is stabilized and bottled.

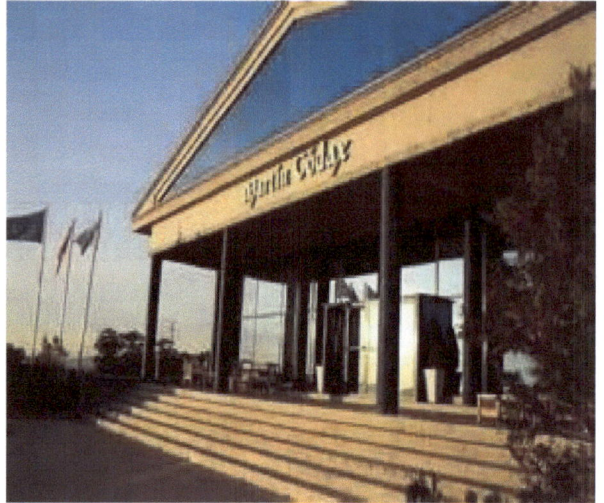

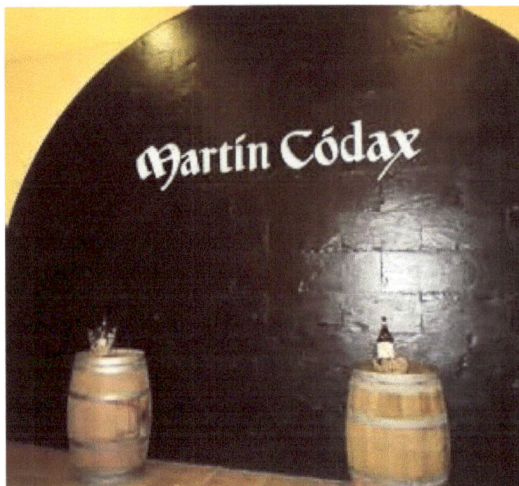

It is generally recommended to enjoy a Albariño when young, one or two years after the harvest for its enjyment. This is a delicate medium body wine, with a festive and crushing finale. Highly aromatic, it brings to the palate notes of apple, peaches, pear and lemon skin, framed in a mineral and spicy touch.

For a perfect mariage, enjoy Martin Códax with seasonal seafood. Due to its minerality and deep acidity, the wine matches perfectly with all "fruits of the sea", emblematic food of the Rías Baixas region.

His reduced 12.8% alcoholic content helps to caress the palate with a long and silky finale.

An authentic "mental celebration"

132

"PRE AND POST" SPIRITUAL LATIN AMERICA
Its successful viticulture absorption, integrates as well its traditions

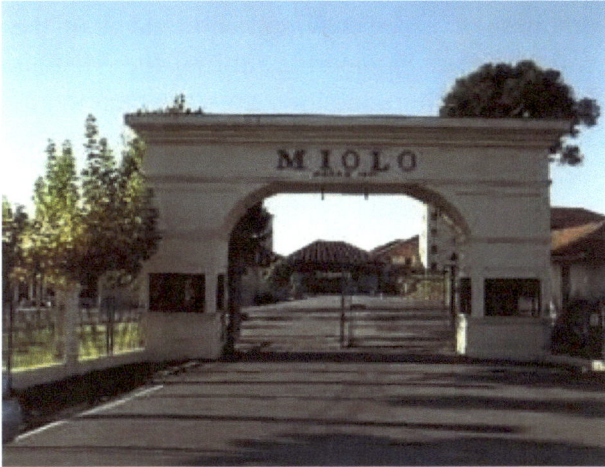

Latin America includes at the present time, as we know, the totallity of the South American Continent, Central America, Mexico and the Caribbean Islands. The similarity among the existing countries, is its common culture, history, language, climate and aspirations of a geopolitical region of greater similarity in our planet. The Catholic Church and its jesuítics ambassadors accompanied the Spanish and Portuguese conquerors in all the trips to the New World bringing with them the Faith in God and the Grapevine, their main Liturgical tool. Between the grapevine cultivation for wine production following Sacramental intentions and European imigrants, it universalized the passage of time opening the wine industry, currently one of the most solid pillars of the Latin American economy.

Nevertheless, the indigenous population of the Pre-Columbian Era, already had an ancestral history of shining political, social and cultural traditions that went back to thousands of years. The creative pleasant drinking sources were also the rites of their diverse religions, as an offer to their Gods, taking place in political and social celebrations, known today as Folklore.

From Northern Mexico to Patagonia, in the South Pole, the fermentation process of fruits and vegetables was widely practiced.

It was of common knowledge that sweet tropical fruits, certain herbs, plants or roots with a natural sugar content, combined with a source of certain bacteria existing in their botanical structure, once macerated with a small dose of pure water, produced an aromatic and relaxing beverage, with a low alcohol content. One of the most popular, during the *Aztec* and *Mayan* Empires was the *pulque,* a sweet beerlike beverage originated from the heart of the *agave* or *maguey*, which continues being consumed nowadays. However, a documented record exists of the first distilled beverage of America. During a catastrophic electrical storm in the Jalisco Valley in Mexico, the heart of the agave was struck by a succession of electrical phenomena providing an unusual heat, creating a distillation process of high alcoholic content. The Aztecs name it *Tequila*, in their language, "Gift of the Gods". Little documentation exists on the fermented types and styles of pre-Columbian beverages, but the finding of amphoras and containing devices in Teotihuacán, Matchu-Pitchu, Monte Albán and other monumental urban and religious centers, demonstrates the existence of "drink for pleasure".

The arrival of the grapevine, followed by its corresponding production process for the production of wine, helped by an emigration without precedents, opened a new sociocultural and industrial stage that, in a

133

long term, would be instrumental in developping a lifestyle transformation. Argentina and the Chilean valleys, with their suitable climatic conditions, are today the front of the production in Latin America and, statistically, they are among the ten greatest countries of viticulture contribution in the world. Other areas, such as Brazil, Uruguay and Peru have been added to the production of wine, but without enjoying convenient microclimates.

At the beginning of the XVI century the *"spirit"* made its appearance in the New Continent: the distillation process. Discovered in the Middle East from immemorial times and introduced in the European Royal Courts by the great physicist and alchemist Michel Savonarola, during the Medicis Renaissance time. Its formula expanded without limits. This phenomenon, together with the creation of the Brandy in the Netherlands, was adopted by the Spanish conquerors. Fruits, grass, roots, flowers and sugar cane were susceptible of being transformed from fermentation to distillation simply increasing a pure water dose while setting a high heat. The resulting steam gave the "spirit " of the dominant ingredient, with a high alcoholic content.

The number of distills depended on the creativity of the indigenous population: *Tequila, Mezcal, Bacanora, Raicilla* and *Charanda* in Mexico. *Pisco* and *Konchak* in Peru and Chile. *Rum* in Puerto Rico, Cuba, Venezuela and sorrounding areas. The *Rum* with exotic species dominated the Antilles. *Brandy* in Colombia and Santo Domingo. And most important to date: the domestic-related distillations that can be enjoyed, at the present time, in all of Latin America regions.

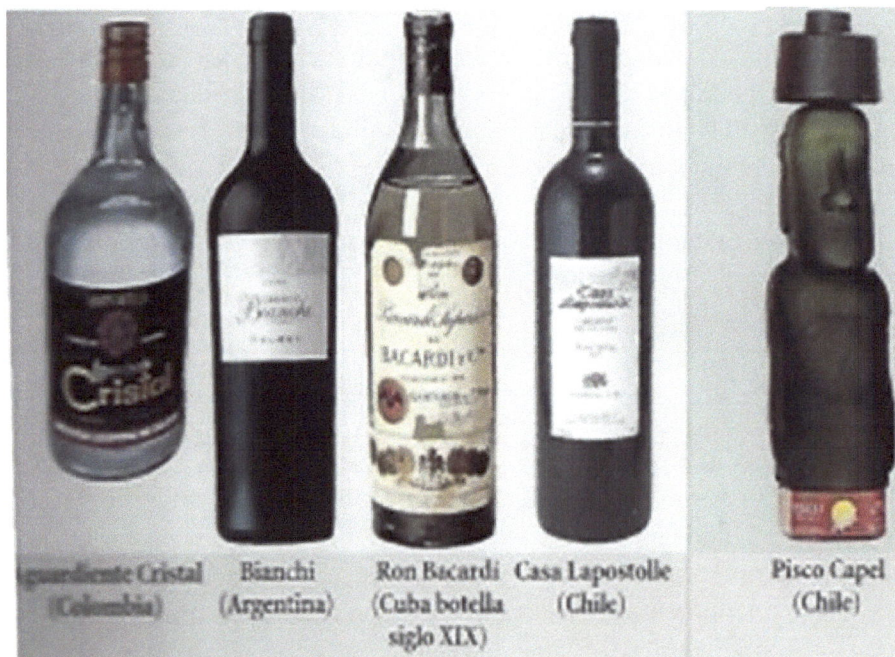

Aguardiente Cristal (Colombia) Bianchi (Argentina) Ron Bacardi (Cuba botella siglo XIX) Casa Lapostolle (Chile) Pisco Capel (Chile)

"LA VIE EN ROSE"
"… EVERYTHING IS IN ACCORDANCE TO THE COLOR OF THE CRYSTAL YOU LOOK THROUGH"

In the times when the Lovers celebrate the hit of Cupid's flying arrows, is most opportune to offer tribute to Rosé Wines, excellent for the table and the "copeo". With exception of the viticulture professionals and isolated fans, the origin, history, elaboration and characteristics of the Rosé Wine are ignored by the consumer in the United States and even in certain European countries.

In the world of love celebrations, Champagnes and all sorts of sparklings are more popular than table wines, which are relegated to second options. This is exactly the opposite to what the historical chronicles affirm. The Greeks are credited with the appearance of the Rosé Wine, fruit of the tempering Mediterranean climate, being the one of more ancestry and quality, coming from Provence, in the south of France. The poet *Homer* relates in *"The Iliad"* the offerings of pink nectars to Jupiter and Aphrodite, goddess of Love. *Herodoto* makes numerous references in its History Treaties to the sweet juice of the Mediterranean grapes. *Terpsícore*, the *muse* of Music and Poetry appeared in multiple murals decanting the pink nectar. However, the red wines never enjoyed a presence in *Mount Olympus*. The elaboration of Rosé Wine differs from the conventional methods due to the acquisition of its color. People generally believe these wines come from a mix of red and white grapes. Nothing is further from the truth! The red grapes along with the skins are squeezed for the fermentation process. The skin begins to color the wine until the desired appearance is obtained. It takes only hours or days to achieve the depth in the color one is looking for. Next, the skins are removed, starting again the traditional method of fermentation.

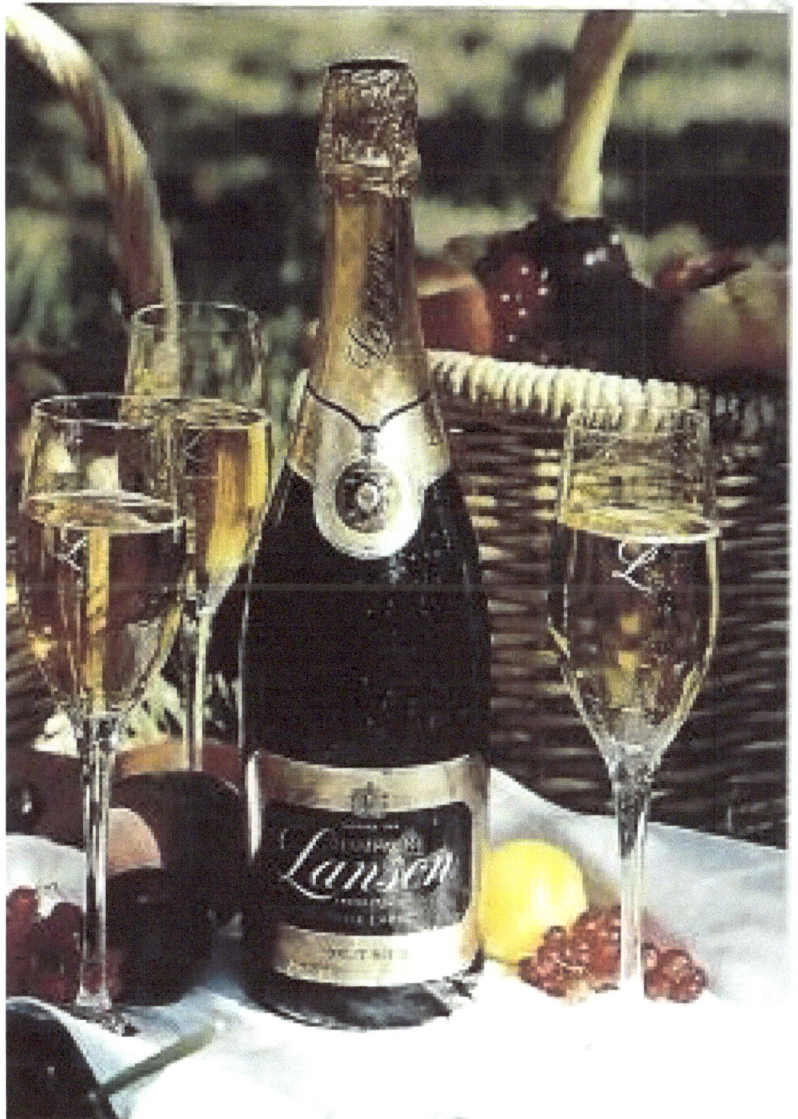

The Rosé Wine must be cosumed when fresh and young, being ideal for *copeo* in temperate climates, accompanying wonderfully the Mediterranean kitchen. Rosé Champagnes, specifically, provide a romantic ambiance to an intimate supper.

FRENCH CHAMPAGNE AND ROSÉ TABLE WINES :

Krug, Louis Roederer Cristal, Dom Perignon, Laurent-Perrier, Veuve Clicquot, Pol Roger and Moet & Chandon, among others, are the most traditionally recognized in the market. However, there are other, not so popular Rosé Champagnes, but of high quality and reasonable price. As far as table wines, remember these names: *Rosé D' Anjou*, with a light sweet taste, *Rosé Tavel*, a velvety dry elixir and the most appreciated, *Cotes de Provence*, of unique style.

"CAVAS" AND SPANISH SPARKLINGS: a great option to enjoy the quality taking advantage of its intrinsic value. *Cava del Penedés"*, produced under the French *Méthode Champenoise* in the *Penedés* Spanish region brings this wine among the finest sparklings in the world. We recommend the *House of Freixenet* presenting soft and dry *Cavas* with a ripe cherry and strawberry pleasant taste.

CALIFORNIA SPARKLING: The most prestigious European wineries have years producing sparkling wines in California. We recommend *Chandon Blanc de Noirs, Etoile Rosé, Louis Roederer Estate Rosé, Pacific Echo of Clicquot* and fabulous *Gloria Ferrer Brut Rosé*, a master blend of Pinot Noir and Chardonnay. Enjoy also the *Gloria Ferrer, Blanc de Noir* with aromas of wild strawberry and black cherry and a fine touch of vanilla.

Worthy of mention are also the Italian *Prosecco, Franzia Corta* and *Asti Spumante.*

Congratulations to all Lovers!

"BEAUJOLAIS NOUVEAU"
The "Old Style" pays a visit as "New" every year

For a few years, in the the great Chef Paul Bocuse Restaurant in Collonges, the famous dancer and coreographer Gene Kelly, with a group of friends, enjoyed the House culinary creations. It was the 21st. of November and everybody was ready to savor the Beaujolais Nouveau of the year. Once served in its "Burgundy" glass, was tasted with curiosity and one of the guests commented, "this wine could have waited for one more week". Gene answered with its special smile: "Perhaps it can, but I don't. The wine is like a dancer in action, he must move with infinite flexibility".

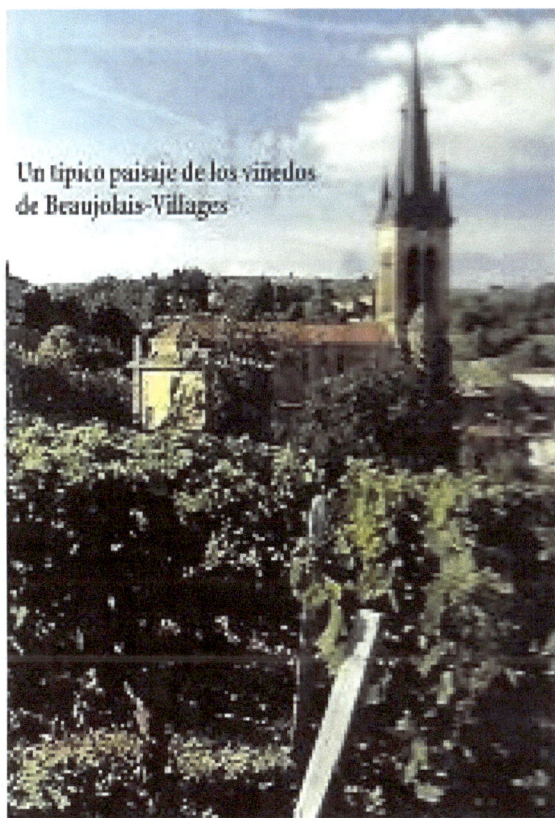

Un tipico paisaje de los viñedos de Beaujolais-Villages

Man did not know how to protect wine from oxidation. Considering that the bottle and the cork, principle of the the wine aging, have less than three hundred years of history, the wine was preserved in wooden barrels, large leather bags or amphoras allowing the contact with oxygen, and, subsequently, turning it in vinegar. From its first Biblical record of existence attributed to Noah (Génesis 9:20), to the end of the XVII century, only the wine of the year was consumed. In 1951 France renewed this custom opening its doors to the Beaujolais trade, a región south of Burgundy, well recognized for its aromatic wines, resting in India Berries flavor making it deliciously easy to drink.

The Beaujolais Nouveau appeared in the world-wide market on the 3rd. thursday of November of every year, its best moment. You must drink it fresh (46 - 54 degrees Fahrenheit), staying in a good shape until the end of January. Although there is no expiration date some could hold a rather longer life. This is a highly anticipated wine carrying a spirit of joy and romanticism.

60% of the Beaujolais Nouveau production is exclusively for Export. In the United States its arrival is an event for the wine lover and all those surrounding the Industry: Hotels, Restaurants, Supermarkets and Liquor Stores.

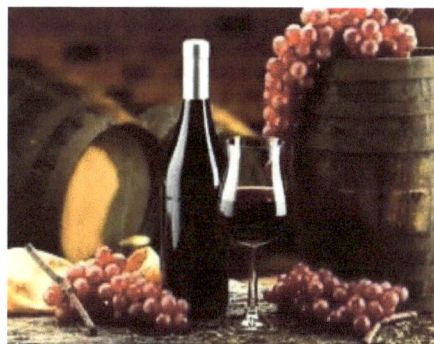

We recommend the following brands: "Georges Duboeuf", consistently awarded for its excellence and freshness, "Barton& Guestier", "Bouchard Pére&Fils", Maison Nicolas","Louis Latour" and "Labouré-Roi". All the "Nouveaus" carry a very reasonable price and is the ideal wine for all types of celebrations, because it goes with infinite menu styles for its lightness and freshness.

Enjoy a "Nouveau" for a modern living!

THE WINES OF "THE RING OF FIRE"
A WASHINGTON STATE PRODIGY

It is necessary to know well the United States North West geography to understand why Washington State is the second wine producer in North America, after California, in volume and quality. Being a link in the geological phenomenon, "The Great Ring of Fire" thus denominated by its volcanic and seismic activity, is now almost inactive and divided by the Cascade mountains.

The west area of the mountain range, following the coastal line, is totally dominated by vigorous marine airflows, translated in frequent and intense rains, very stormy skies, cold temperatures and high atmospheric humidity. All these factors disable the cultivation of the grapevine. Nevertheless, by the east of the mountain range, is the Columbia Valley, considered a "garden" for grape development and optimal wine production. The Columbia, Snake and Yakima rivers, irrigate a rich subsoil shaped by volcanic and basaltic crests. Its low humidity climate, intense sunlight and warm temperature, together with a long European tradition in winemaking since 1871, provides the suitable elements for the production of an extraordinary variety of wines of the highest quality, from Rieslings to Syrahs. In a "blind tasting" for professionals, recently carried out in Miami , three wines of the State of Washington received higher marks than Château Mouton Rothschild and Caymus. Of the 300 vineyards currently existing we have selected:

CHÂTEAU STE. MICHELLE:

In 1871, missionaries and leather retailers brought from France in their trips to Washington State fresh plantings and seeds of the grapevine variety "Grenache", teaching the Native Americans how to build diversifying irrigation channels from the Yakima river. In 1912, Frederick Stimson, a recognized industrialist, founded a commercial conglomerate for table wine elaboration by the northeast of Seattle, building a *Palacete* surrounded by exotic gardens which are included in the National Historical Places Registry. Its first produced wine: **Château Ste. Michelle**. Mr. Stimson's dream has been incredibly surpassed. Château Ste. Michelle at the moment produces a wine diversity of great consistency due to the climate changes, the *terroir* wealth, a total plague absence and a wise technology.

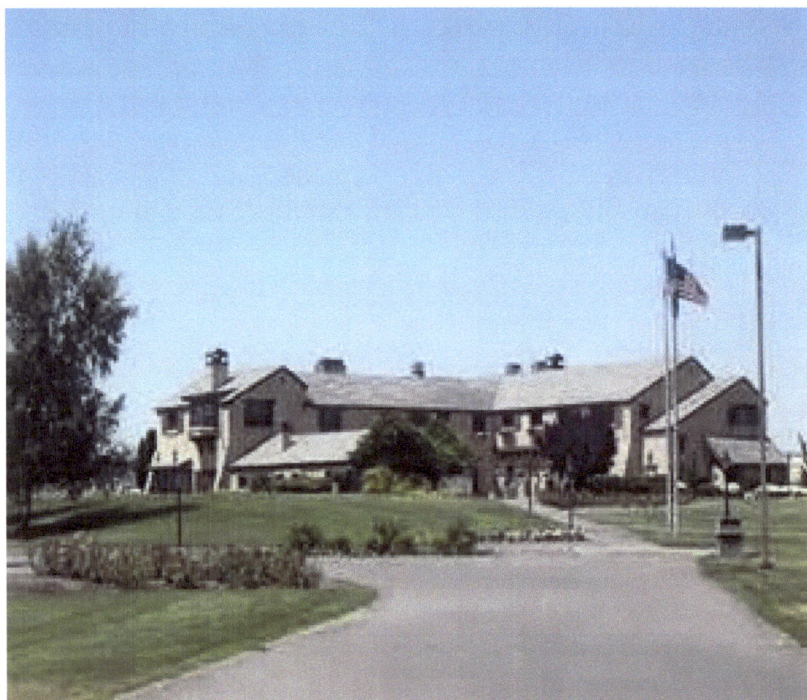

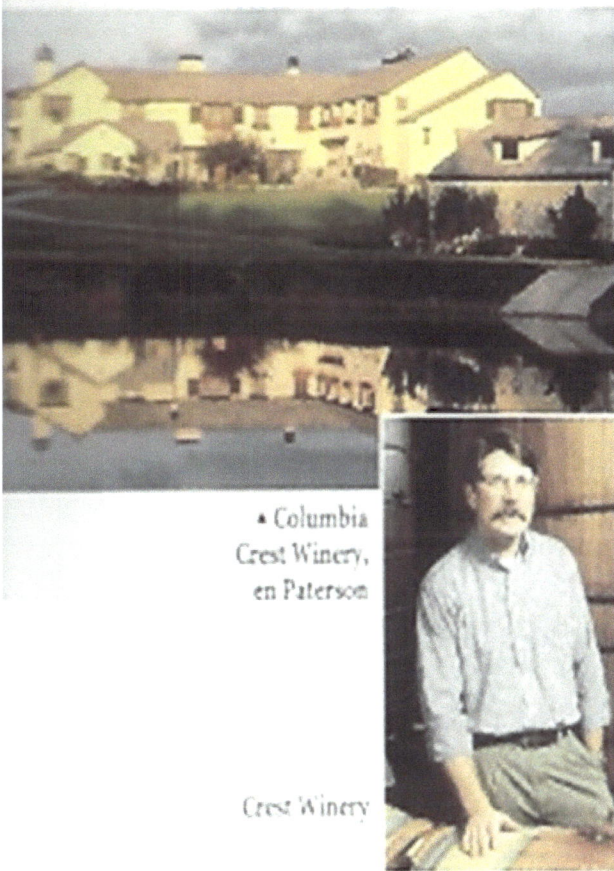

Columbia Crest Winery, en Paterson

Crest Winery

Wine Production: Gewurztraminer - Johannisberger Riesling - Gray Pinot - Sauvignon Blanc-Semillon - Chardonnay (exceptional) - Merlot - Cabernet Sauvignon - Riesling - Syrah-Hoist Wine Reserve - Artist Meritage Series (hand painted labels).

COLUMBIA CREST:

Born in 1978 and being one of the Washington State most recent wineries, **Columbia Crest** conquered the market based on technology and the art of European style winemaking. In 1979, at a cost of $26 million dollars, a European Chateau is built in Paterson, the Southeastern end of the State, near the Oregon border, lodging Columbia Crest.

Perhaps it could be called an "obtained miracle", but in reality all its profits have been fruit of a great industrial vision, based on producing and offering the best wines at a popular cost. Wine Production: Johannisberger Riesling - Gewurztraminer - Sauvignon Blanc - Semillon - Chardonnay - Semillon Chardonnay – Merlot, a 1994 Gold medal in Bordeaux - Syrah - Cabernet Sauvignon.

DOMAINE STE. MICHELLE:

Located in the heart of the Columbia Valley, the vineyard is dedicated exclusively to the production of Sparkling Method wines, delicately articulating the four Champagne aromas: Cuvée Brut, Blanc de Blancs, Blanc de Noir and Extra Dry.

To all wine lovers: Visit the State of Washington, especially in the summer months!

MANZANILLA: THE MISCHIEVOUS ANDALUSIAN GOBLIN
A charming "wine spell"

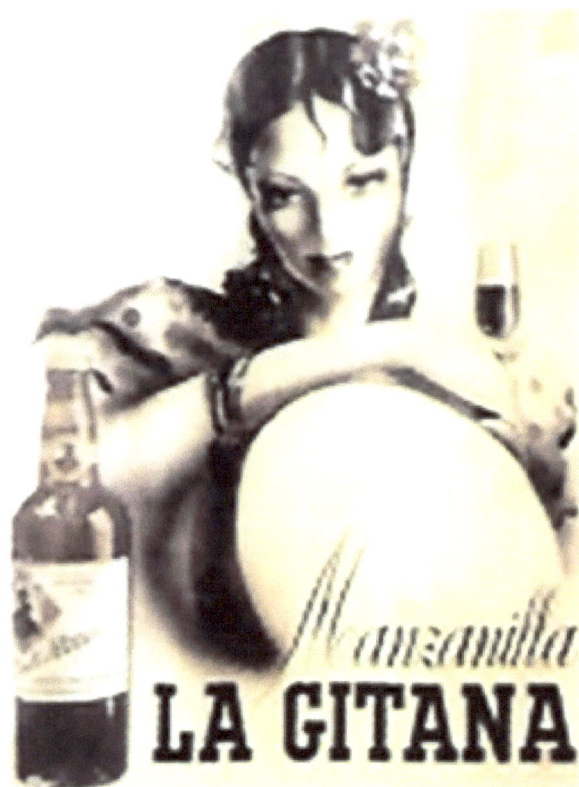

A few miles from *Jerez de La Frontera*, where the *Guadalquivir* river spills its waters and Andalusian history in the Atlantic Ocean, vibrates the enchanted town of *Sanlúcar de Barrameda*, were Manzanilla was born. Pale, dry and light, this "naughty" wine, was elaborated to raise the joy in happy drinking palates.

This area, resting between the shore and the sea, gives rise to a smooth microclimate with a constant humidity, allowing the growth and permanence of living "*fungi*" or "*flor*", protecting the wine, a type of Sherry, from oxidation, turning it in a higher quality elixir. Its special sea-environment of a unique character among Sherry wines, brings the Manzanilla to the top the wine world.

To open a bottle of Manzanilla is a prelude to friendship, a feast, good humor and a great contagious joy, locking up the spirit of Andalusia. Drink it fresh and is ideal to accompany *tapas* and seafood, or to integrate it in a good Garlic Soup. Is also the heart of the *Andalusian Gazpacho*.

Nowadays Manzanilla is practically consumed as a table wine, putting a rejoicing accent in the daily supper. A great example of grape growing lineage points to the "Hidalgo Winery of Sanlúcar de Barrameda", founded in 1792 by Don José Pantaleón Hidalgo, with the appearance of *Manzanilla* in the market, the product considered to date as the pride of the family. In the XIX century, under the direction of his son Don Eduardo Hidalgo, the winery became involved in the production of all types of Sherry wines: *"Fino", "Amontillado", "Palo Cortado"," Oloroso", "Raya"* and *"Pedro Ximénez"*, in addition to brandys *"Solera Gran Reserva"*. Nevertheless, the favorite daughter was always the *Manzanilla*, which he named *"La Gitana"* or "The Gipsy Girl" in English.

In the middle of the century "Hidalgo House" had obtained numerous awards in exhibitions and International contests, exporting its wines to the United States, firstly in barrels of American Oak, later bottled. Currently, Manzanilla "La Gitana" is the most popular in the Spanish market, being the preferred wine of the city of *Sevilla*, the heart of Andalusia.

140

RAIN OF GOLD IN JEREZ

The glorious Spanish Brandy among the Spirts Industry

The root of the English word "Brandy" comes originally from the Dutch, *branden* (the spirit) or *brandewijn* (Brandy Wine). Only two Brandy producing regions exist presently in the world under Denomination of Origin: "Cognac" - French province of Charente Armagnac and *"Jerez de la Frontera"* in Andalusia, in southwest Spain. The rich and chalky Andalutian *terroir*, bathed by the the Mediterranean Sea waters and the Atlantic Ocean, creates a unique combination leading to the production of some of the greatest "Solera Gran Reserva" brandys in the world.

The *"Jerez"* grape growers, since 1483, settled down the pertinent regulations for the control and authentication of its fermentation and distillation process of its wines and spirits, ratified internationally in 1891, year in which was born the *Jerez* Denomination of Origin.

The *Gran Duque de Alba Brandy, Solera Gran Reserva*, recently winner of two gold medals granted by the **2008 San Francisco World Spirits Competition** and the **Beverage Testing Institute's International Review of Spirits**, in London, is produced by the renowned Williams & Humbert *Bodegas de Jerez*, certified as the largest in the world, possessing 1,200 hectares of vineyards. When analyzing the labels of the finest "Jerez" brandies, we appreciate that many are baptized with Monarchs names such a Carlos I, Philip II, Carlos III, members of the Spanish Royalty, Duque de Alba, Cardenal Mendoza and heroic events of great historic value, such as the Battle of Lepanto, and the Independence War. In this way, the highest lineage *bodegas* compared their products with the top aristocratic elite, reflected in centuries of the History of Spain. Fernando Alvarez de Toledo, *Duque de Alba*, brave soldier and astute Man of State, stood out under the Carlos V reign as a military and political genius that, with the conquest of Portugal and the Netherlands, took the *Austrias Dinasty* to its pinacle. The brandy *Gran Duque de Alba* carefully ages around 12 years in oak barrels under the system *"Solera"*, uniquely Spanish, who is also used for the Sherry Wines of more style in the world. Its gold-mahogany color is a spectacle of Mother Nature. Aromas of toasted nuts, caramel, dark fruits and a smooth touch of spice gives the palate a smooth finale. Enjoy it at room temperature in a snifter after an egregious supper. Also ideal with creative desserts. The Williams&Humbert *bodega* just launched a new product into the United States, the *Crema de Alba*, winner of a Silver Medal in the above mentioned competitions. A delicious creamy liqueur with aromas of vanilla and cocoa. Drink it on ice or simply cold in a cordial glass. Fascinating!

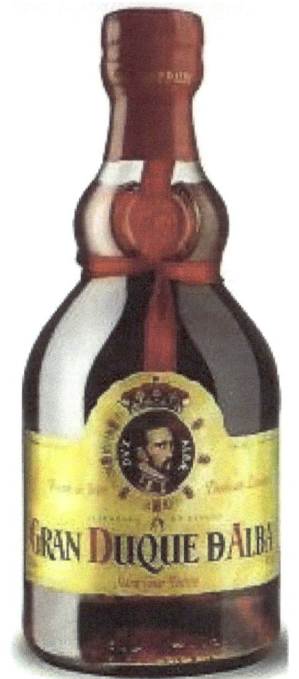

"Viva Jerez y la Tierra Andaluza" !

THE SCIENCE OF THE SPIRITS
"Cocktail". The art of Mixology

In 1786, Martha Washington never conceived that her festive "Rum Punch" would make history. At the time, her husband George was the founder of the " Great Distillery of Mount Vernon" and President of the United States of America. Their family blend was going to be a part of a new study about a compatible distills mixture of sweet "liqueurs" , numerous varieties of fruits, wild herbal scents and exotic spices. He called it "Mixology". Today, 219 years later, more than 9.000 combined spirits or "cocktails" are registered in the "International Mixologists Guild" in London.

With a few tentative exceptions, light punches resulting from mixing certain wines and citrus, macerated with fruit, *acqua vitae* or Rum of the Islands, were consumed pure until the end of the XVIII century. Adding any other ingredients besides a noble Cognac, an illustrious Whiskey or Wines of aristocratic origin, was described as an adultery. The mid 1800s marked the birth of the "Cocktail Era" in America, but it was the XX century, without a doubt, the "Golden Cocktail Time", settling mainly in the feminine sector, smooth and artistic alternatives for the distills enjoyment.

The "Cocktail" influence in a new "social life style" lasts to present times. It should be served cold. We attended "cocktail parties". The ladies shine in "cocktail dresses". We share with friends in the bar to the heat of a "cocktail". We began supper with a "cocktail" we created with pride. We fight against daily pressure savoring a "cocktail".

We enjoy vacations sipping good "tropical cocktails". We ordered in the restaurant gastronomical combinations like "cocktail of…" and, definitively,…"life is cocktail and love", melodic line of a Carlos Gardel popular tango Singer, and, 19 years of Prohibition (1919-1933) did not make an impression in "Mixology" development. Mary Sondergaard, an adventurous "New York Society" millionaire of the 1920s. , great lover of transatlantic cruise trips, expended time and time again thinking about how to fill the vacuum between the "Tea Time" and "Supper". During one of her trips New York- Paris, she became a close friend of Fernand Petiot, a nice and creative American, Head of Barmans on the cruise-ship "Ile-de-France".

Using his "great host virtues", he introduced for the passengers recreation "The Cocktail Hour", becoming fashionable among the European society and a favorite "American Dusk" pastime. At the end of fthe 20s, Mary found Fernand again, as a barman of *"Harry' s New York Bar"* in Paris. Knowing Miss Sondergaard was suffering from a severe "hangover", Fernand assured her that his last creation "would help a lot" to releave her hardship. "I will baptise this cocktail with your name".

It worked! "The Bloody Mary" was born. It is the talent and creativity of the "Fernands" of the world what makes of Mixology a science of contributing factors, increasing the sensual wealth of the individual.

"THE MARTHA WASHINGTON" PUNCH   (Serves 6 – 10)
Ingredients

3 oz. White Rum   3 Sliced in quarts Lemons
3 oz. Aged Rum   1 Sliced in quarts Orange
4 oz. Orange Couracao   ½ Nutmeg teaspoon
4 oz. White Syrup   3 Crushed Cinnamon Sticks
4 oz. Fresh Lemon Juice   6 Cloves
4 oz. Fresh Orange Juice   12 oz. Boiling Water

PROCEDURE: Mix lemons and oranges with cinnamon, clove and nutmeg until achieving under fire a homogenous mass. Add white syrup, lemon and orange juice to the boiling water. Let it get to room temperature and steer the mixture with rums and orange couracao. Strain in a crystal container, adding ice. Decorate with orange slices, lemon branches and cinnamon sticks, dusting ground nutmeg on top.

First President. First "Cocktail Maker"!

THE GREAT WOMEN INFLUENCE IN OUR INDUSTRY
Today's outstanding Gallery

The existing *"Taboo"* until the beginning of the XX century, referring to Women participation in the world of the politics and business, collapsed with great noise when in August of 1920 the United States of America modified the 19th. Amendment of the Constitution declaring: "The right to vote of the United States citizens can not be denied nor limited by the Federal Government due to sexual identity". This was the first integration passage, an example of most countries governed under Democracy.

In the Western World most agricultural works were traditionally trusted to the feminine hand, due to the numerous field work, especially in the grape growing scope, vineyard planting, fertilizing, harvesting, stepped crushing and filtration, until mechanic processes changed the wine production routine. Once fulfilling these tasks, the man was in charge of the intricate process of carrying out the fermentation, mixing, maturing, bottling and labeling, administrative direction and product sales. These barriers and limitations no longer exist today. Women can presently carry out, in many cases with matchless efficiency, the tasks attributed exclusively to men by centuries.

57% of the wine sold in the United States are acquired by women, being the majority of decision taking over what wines move better in the Market, setting the new century trajectory. From reaching excellence in winemaking or spirit distilling, to carrying out deserved positions, such as Presidents and C.E.O.s of millionaire companies, women are involved in the front of the International Wine Market business and are also, without a doubt, in Marketing, Communications and Public Relations.

 I present for our readers, in a brief gallery, a few images of illustrious women pertaining to our Industry And we also want to add the following Honorary Mentions:

Margareth Henríquez- President. HOUSE OF KRUG Champagne
Marimar Torres, owner of "MARIMAR" WINERY (Sonoma), pioneer of THE ORGANIC METHOD.
Eva Bertrán, Executive Vicepresident, FREIXENET / SEGURA VIUDAS / GLORIA FERRER.
Robin Pollard, Executive Director. WASHINGTON WINE COMMISSION.
Amelia Durand – Communications Director, MOET HENNESSY USA.
Whitley Bouma y **Camille Broderick**, International Ambassadors, MOET- HENNESSY USA.

"And many many more".

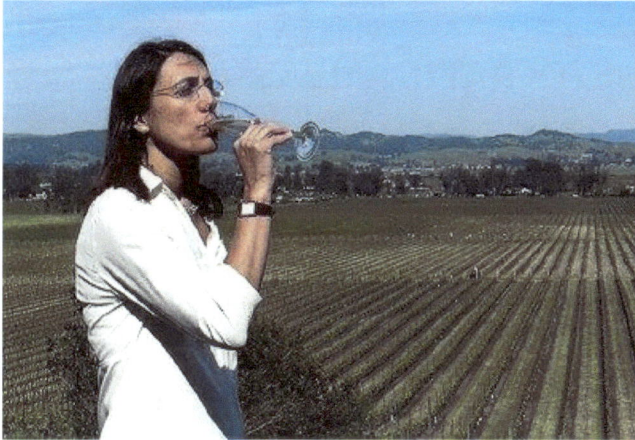

Eva Beltrán

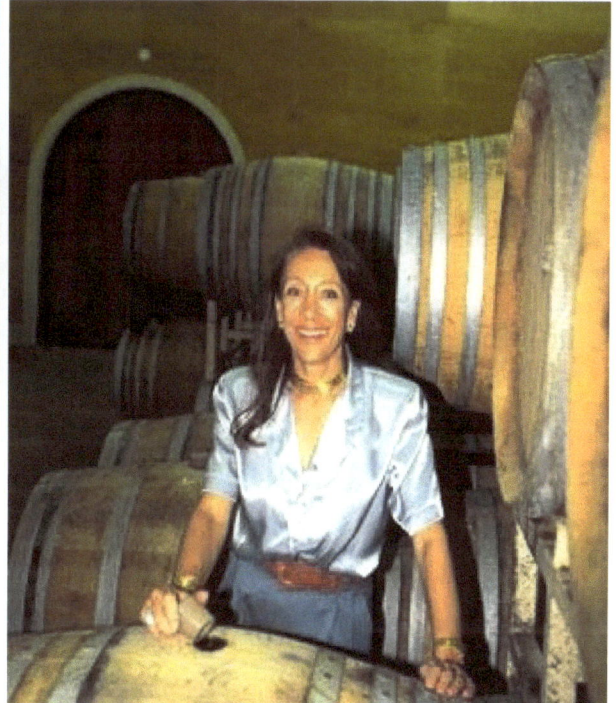

Marimar Torres,

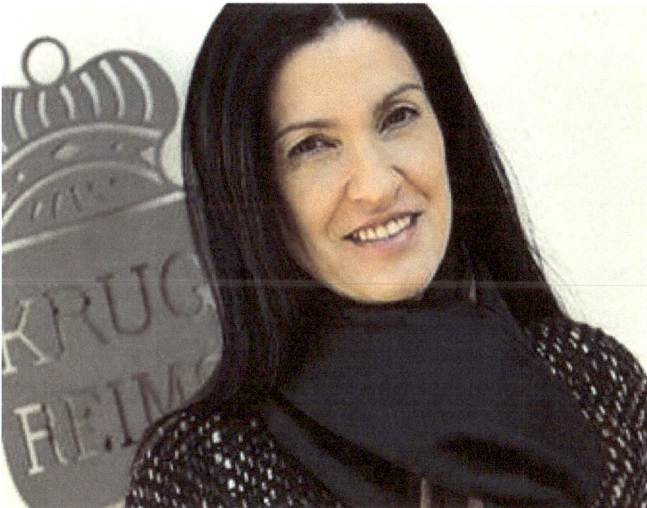

Margareth Henríquez

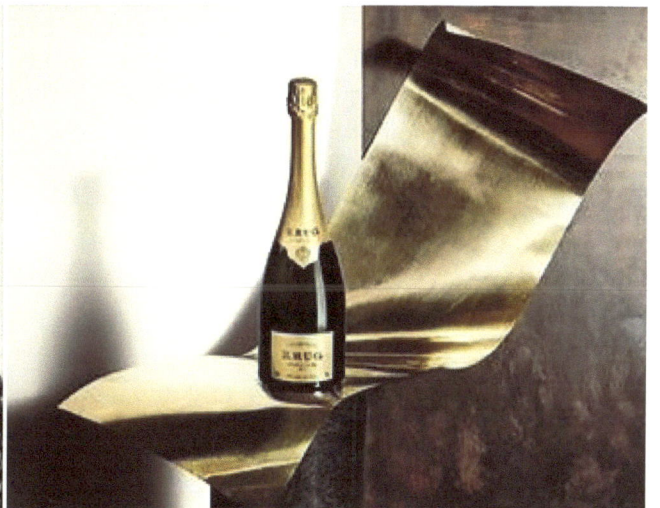

THE *"RIBERA DEL DUERO"* ARISTOCRATIC AMBASSADOR
"Vega Sicilia", The Great

"Bodegas Vega Sicilia" offers a forceful example of tenacity before adversity in the world-wide Wine Industry. It was in 1859 when Don Eloy Lecanda received from his father a 2,000 hectares property in the Castilian *plateaux*, bordering the *Duero* river. By the year 1880 this immense property became an "Agricultural Empire" in Spain. Aside from also being a fine cattle ranch, a source of fruits and an artistic folkloric ceramics nest, Don Eloy imported from Bordeaux thousands of stocks and plantings of Cabernet Sauvignon, Merlot, Carmènere, Malbec and Pinot Noir. With a noble visionary intention for wine production, he assigned 150 hectares of the property, at more than 700 meters of altitude by the river borders, with a perfect microclimate.

The Spanish Wine mythology was born in the fertile Vega Sicilia and Carrascal valleys. Nevertheless, Don Eloy, as it happened to his father, was not able to face his financial obligations. After fifteen years of misfortune, a *philoxera* plague in La Rioja and a multitude of corporative intrigues, the Lecanda business changed its name to *"Antonio Herrero & Sons"*, owners of a successful *Bodega* in La Rioja. The worldly temperament and the sweeping personality of these brothers, cosmopolitan and well related, were instrumental in producing a different wine, to maintain the business image of the family.

Between 1915 and 1917, under the Herrero family, a red wine of sophisticated technique of maturation and elegant Baroque style was labeled Vega Sicilia Unico. Without a harvesting year, it was sent to the market with the following composition: 70% Tempranillo, 20% Cabernet Sauvignon, 10% Merlot, Malbec and Albillo. It was only produced in perfect years. Versatile, of a dark cherry color, with deep aromas and a unique character of fruit caressed by the *sureño* sun. The result of a bouquet combination of dry fruits, figs, dark plums, wild berries, tobacco, coffee and spices. A work of Art!

Most of the selected production was given out to the European aristocracy without financial profit. Obviously, to cover the financial holes, the Vega Sicilia Unico became the most expensive wine of Spain. Simply, it was a wine that could not be bought only with money but mainly with friendship. Meanwhile, the Ribera del Duero region, in the hands of cooperatives and wine merchants, produced in numerous amounts, simple and honest red wines for table and copeo consumption supplying Madrid, only within a distance of 200 miles encompassing the local business areas. The company changed hands several times, until in 1982 was acquired by the Alvarez family, heading the great Vega Sicilia business.

"There are wines created by its owners and owners elevated to the glory by certain wines. I represent neither one nor another alternative", affirms Pablo Alvarez responsible for the *bodegas* at the present time. Without letting himself to be dragged by the passion towards the wine nor by its name, he applied rigor and attention to detail the "vegasicilian" microcosm, as if it were a sacred rule. This story can be compared to a past Wall Street tale, crystallized in the present, by four wines produced by the Winery:

"Vega Sicilia Unico Reserva Especial", Vega *Sicilia Cosecha, Valbuena Quinto Año* (named by Don Eloy in honor of his great friend *Marques de Valbuena*) and *Alión*, a most popular wine.

Today, the *Vega Sicilia Unico Reserva Especial,* only sold by allocation, is the favorite red wine of the Royalty and the European Aristocracy and also accompanies the tables of the High Corporate World.

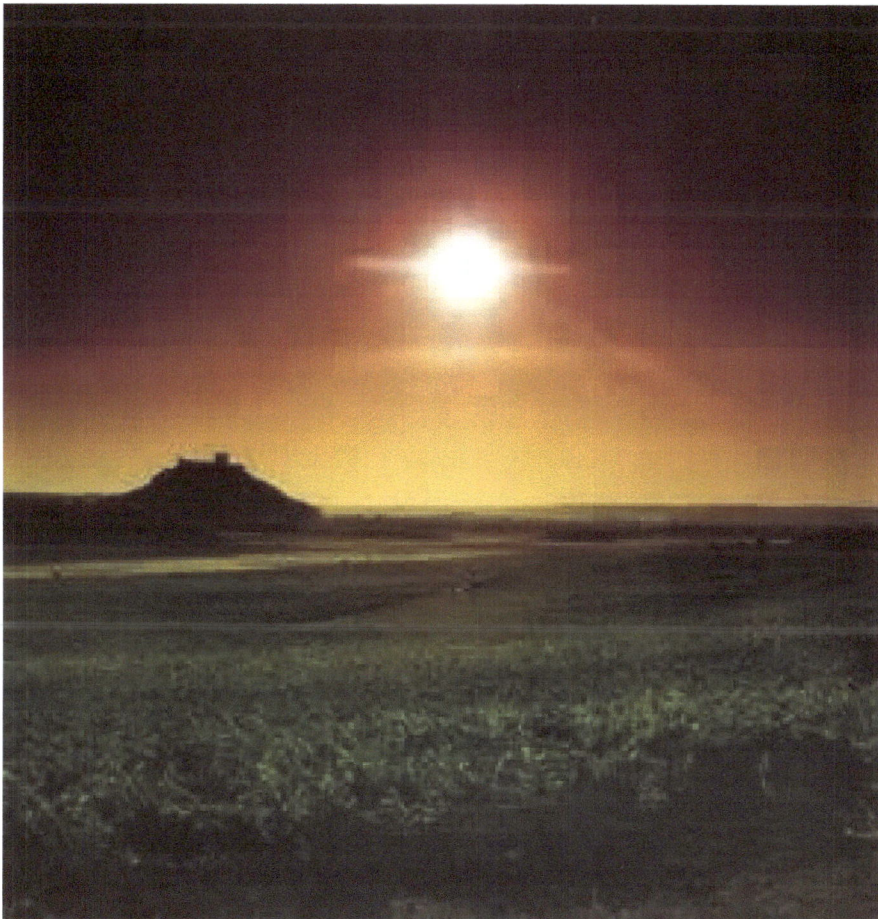

VODKA: SIMPLICITY AND PURITY OF A SPIRIT

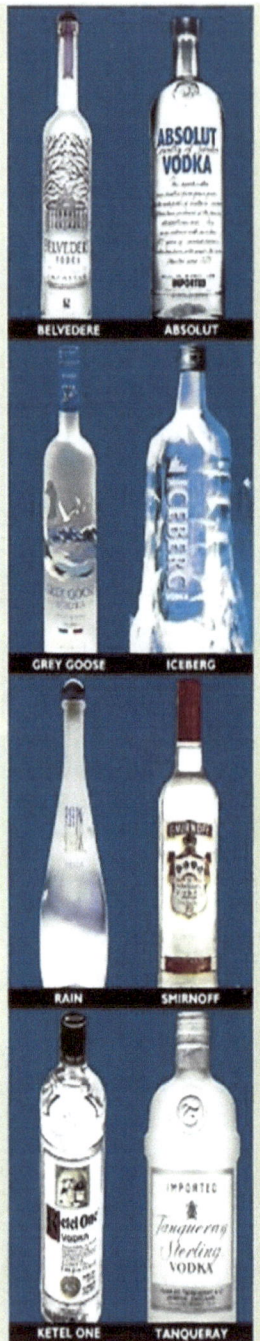

"Vodka" in the Russian language or "Wodka" in Polish, is an affectionate term of the word "water" that could be translated as "little water". Its history goes back to antiquity. To date there is a strong controversy on the discovery of the distilled alcoholic beverage, considered to be the Russian national spirit. Nevertheless Poland claims to be the pioneer of its production going back to the VIII century. On the other hand, there are written accounts by the end of the IX century giving Russia a higher credibility in this eternal discussion. According to "Chronicle of Vyatka" published in 1174, the reality is that the first distillery was founded in the region of Khylnovsk in Russia.

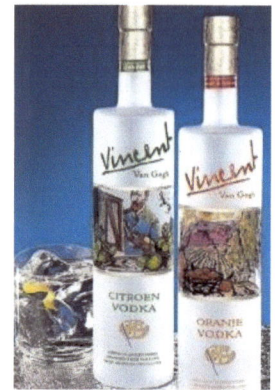

During the Middle Ages, Vodka was used largerly for medicinal purposes as well as in the production of gunpowder. It was until the XIV century when the Vodka formally was considered a "drink".

The first distilleries began producing the "spirit", using most of the abundant agricultural fruits in the regions: wheat, rye, corn, potatoes, sugar beet or the combination of several of these products which are to date, the base of its distillation. Successively, the mass was filtered through vegetal coal layers adding pure water, considered the most important ingredient in Vodka. As the production increased, began the exports from Russia and Poland, penetrating in the neighboring western Kingdoms and Royal Courts. In the mid XIV century, Sir Douglas Hume, English Ambassador to Moscow, described the Vodka as the Russian national drink and in the XVI century, Poland, Finland and the present Baltic countries characterized it as their own spirit "par excellence". The result of this "fight" was the exotic prestige of a perfect "liqueur", with no specific flavor, of high concentration and unusual smoothness.

At the beginning of the XIX century, due to the Napoleonic Wars, the demand of Vodka grew enormously for "the soldiers consumption". By the end of this century, with standard techniques of production and quality assurance, the name "Vodka" was officially recognized. After the Russian Revolution in 1918, the Bolshevik government confiscated all private distilleries causing a migratory wave of vodka producers that settled down in diverse European countries. In 1934, in Paris, the first Vodka distillery of the western world appeared, Smirnoff, acquired by a North American company in 1946. Then the vodka began to conquer the western market with a success without precedent. Presently, one of four bottles of licor consumed in the United States is Vodka. Its compatibility of combination and mixes is amazing due to the deficiency of a specific flavor without producing buccal stench. From the 90s. beginning, endless number of innovations in distillation techniques, exotic flavors and aromas, bottle designs and bitter competition in marketing research methods, has done of Vodka the distilled of more consumption throughout the world, produced in the five continents. The ideal style to tasting Vodka is straight, at freezing temperature in fine crystal glass of a one ounce average. The Vodka Martini is number one in popularity in a large list of world-wide coctails, surpassing the Gin as the basic ngredient. Let's name the most outstanding vodkas in our Market:

ABSOLUT: Sweden.
ICEBERG: Canada.
GREY GOOSE: France.
KETEL ONE: Holand.
VINCENT Van Gogh: Holand.
BELVEDERE: Poland.
CHOPIN: Poland.
CIROC: France, grape distilled.
RAIN: U.S.A. Organic grain.
SMIRNOFF: U.S.A. ideal for mixing.
STOLICHNAYA: Rusia. Traditional.
FINLANDIA: Escandinavia.
VOX: Holand.
PEARL: Canada.
TANQUERAY STERLING: England.
ULTIMAT: Poland

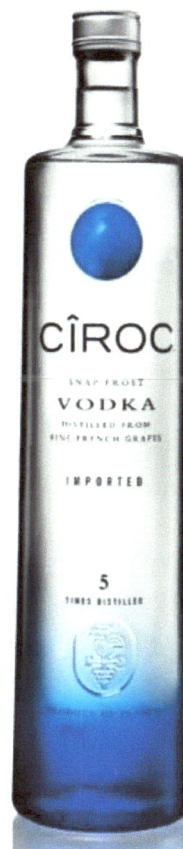

THE PROGRESSIVE WINE INDUSTRY OF MODERN CHILE

A more illustrious route of its fertile Valleys and modern Wineries

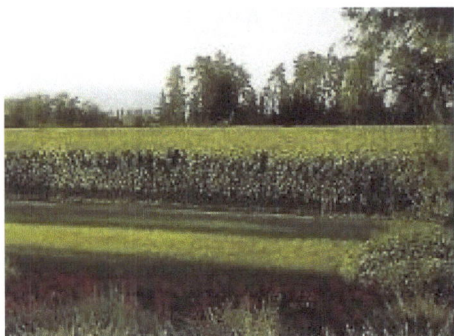

The Chilean climate, especially in the central Valleys, is enviable. Proteged by the Andean mountain range, the soil health, fertility and the organic defense from the *phylloxera* plague, are guaranteed by Mother Nature. In the history of Chilean grape growing, we find an endless number of *Vitis Vinifera* varieties. The pioneer grapes *País* and *Mission*, became the most popular for the elaboration of illoustrious table wines, such as Cabernet Sauvignon, Merlot, Cabernet Franc, Malbec, Pinot Noir, Chardonnay and Sauvignon Blanc among others. Nevertheless, the grape growes searched for a virtuous Grapevine for many years with the necessary characteristics to identify a variety as the Chile's National Grape. Let's mention the *Malbec* from Argentina, the French *Cabernets*, the Italian *Sangiovesse* or the *Tempranillo* from Spain. It recently appeared.. An old *French Bordalesse* variety revived from History offering optimal conditions for cultivation in the Chilean *terroir*: The CARMENERE, also known as Grande Vidure, appearing in the Market as 100% varietal or as integral of wise blends. Carrying a great European influence and Californian technical advance, the following Wineries represent the peak of the wine production of Chile:

Emiliana. Organic Vineyards: The first Winery using this new agricultural technique in Chile. The vine must be deeply planted, forcing it to work hard to detect and absorb its nutrients. **Emiliana** bottles its wines under a single name, **Sincerity,** presenting two varietals, Chardonnay and Sauvignon Blanc, both coming from the *Valle of Casablanca.*
Masterful blends:
Sincerity 2001, 2002, 25% Cabernet Sauvignon – 75% Merlot, *Valle de Rapel.*
Sincerity 2003, 45% Cabernet Sauvignon – 55% Merlot. *Valle de Rapel.*

Casa Lapostolle: Founded in 1994. At present time the company owns 320 hectares, producing a total of 150.000 wine cases. The most distinguished wines are: it is the Clos de Apalta, 85% Carmènere - Merlot, 15% Cabernet Sauvignon, Colchagua/Valley of Rapel. Cuvée denomination Alexandre:
Clos de Apalta, 85% Carmenere, 15% Cabernet Sauvignon-Merlot.*Colchagua-Valle de Rapel*
Chardonnay 2004, 100% Chardonnay. *Valle de Casablanca.*
Cabernet Sauvignon 2003, 85% Cabernet Sauvignon – 15% Merlot. *Valle de Colchagua.*
Syrah 2003, 100% Syrah. *Valle de Rapel.*
Borobo, 35% Pinot Noir, 25% Merlot, 20% Syrah, 10% Cabernet Sauvignon, 10% Carmenère, Casablanca *and Requinoa.*

Viña Montes: The new sensation in the Market. A classic and innovating Winery that launched with aclamation the ***Purple Angel 2003***, 92% Carmènere and 8% Pétit Verdot, along with ***Montes Folly 2003***, 100% Sirah and ***Montes Alpha "M" 2003***, 80% Cabernet Sauvignon, 10% Cabernet Franc, 5% Merlot and 5% Pétit Verdot.

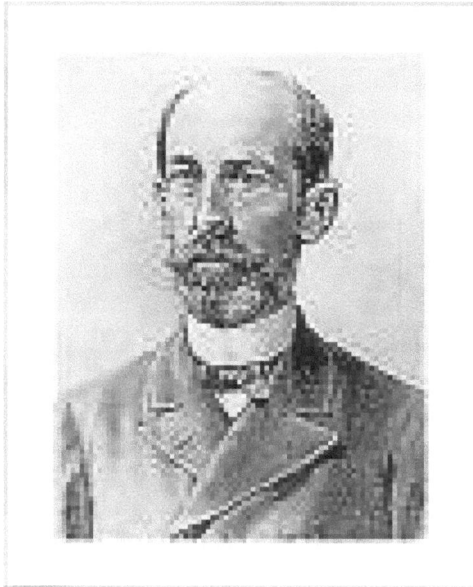

Concha y Toro: In 1833 Don Melchor de Concha y Toro and his wife Emiliana Subercaseaux began importing the finest grapevines of Bordeaux, creating nowadays the more extensive and popular viticultural complex of Chile. The main Winery is based in the Valley of Maipo, its vineyards by The Andes shade.

The *Concha y Toro* wines are defined as follows:
Almaviva (in association with the House Mouton-Rothschild), Amelia, ***Casillero del Diablo, Marqués de Casa Concha, Terrunyo, Trío, Sunrise, Frontera.***
And, a Cabernet Sauvignon of the greatest class in the world: ***Don Melchor***, as a tribute to the Patriarch.

Viña Errázuriz: Perhaps one of the most progressive companies in the Chilean and international Wine World. Established in *Valle Aconcagua* in 1870, its founder, Don Maximiano Errázuriz initiated the plantation of Cabernet Sauvignon, Merlot, Cabernet Franc and Syrah. Among the great wine range produced by the Winery excelles Seña (in association with Robert Mondavi Winery) and ***Don Maximiano Founder's Reserve.   Viñedo Chadwick***.

Veramonte: A modern conglomerate in the *Valle de Casablanca,* built by its proprietor, Agustín Huneeus, grape grower of Napa Valley, that appreciated the similarity between both *terroirs*. Its proximity to Santiago allowed him to add a Visitors Center to the wineries which, nowadays, receives more than 30.000 people at year. The 100% varietal style predominates in the production: Sauvignon Blanc, Chardonnay, Merlot, Cabernet Sauvignon and Primus, Veramonte's expert blend of Carmènere and Cabernet Sauvignon.

Take a trip to Paradise. Don't miss it !

PORTUGAL AND ITS VIBRANT WINES

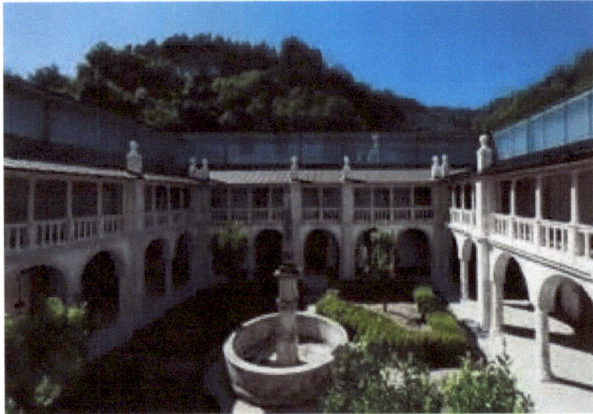

The European Union gave the Welcome to Portugal in 1986, opening the door to one of the oldest nations of the Continent. Constituted as an independent Kingdom in 1143, Portugal is part of the Iberian Peninsula with identical borders that those delimited in 1297. The country was populated, occupied and invaded since early times during a period of 850 years, exposing itself to an eclectic influence of distant Civilizations.

The Celtic settlers, the Phoenician merchants, the Roman Empire, the *Suevos* and *Visigodos* barbarian hordes and the Arab conquest wove an embroider of cultures, rich inheritance of today's Porrtugal. *Lisboa*, the capital, *Oporto*, *Coímbra* and *Bethlehem*, among many other cities, is a proof of it.

Although there is a record of the Monastery of *Lorvao* vineyards, dating from the 950 B.C., the presence of wine becomes real around the year 600 A.C. in which the Phoenicians penetrated in the south of the Iberian Peninsula bringing grape plantings for cultivation with such hability, that have survived by 2.500 years. Four centuries later the Romans extended towards the north occupying the *Valle del Río Duero*, the producing region of the *Oporto*, wine. Cylindrical stones for pressing the grapes and mud amphoras for the wine fermentation and storage, were found in the area. The art of grapevine viticulture and the spiritual elixirs elaboration have not stopped since then. Portugal is recognized anywhere in the world as the unique producer of the wonderful *Oporto* or Port Wine and the fine *Madeira*. Also has multiplied its wine production investments competing highly, contributing with an extraordinary variety of wines of unique and individual character.

Presenting:

VINHO VERDE. *Río Minho* región, producing exclusively white wines of *Loureiro* and *Alvarinho* varieties. A fresh wine of fruity character and low in alcohol (9%-10%).
DOURO. From *Valle del Río Duero*. Red wines product of Touriga *Nacional* and *Fino Malvasia*. Different characters depending on the variety of grape. From balanced and elegant, to powerful, intense color and high tannins.

DAO. From the Atlantic Coast. Red wines of *Roriz* and *Pinheira* grapes of great quality. It ages very well.

BUCELAS. North of Lisbon Valleys. Red wine from *Arinto* grape . Dry with slight acidity. Favorite of George III, George IV, the Duke of Wellington and Thomas Jefferson.

ALENTEJO. Produced in Southeastern región. 50% of the cork of the world comes from this area. White and red wines from Periquita, *Aragonés and Ropeiro* grapes. Complejos, of good, elegant body and great aging process.

They are also worthy of considering these Noble wines:

BAIRRADA COLARES CARCAVELOS TRAS-OS-MONTES BEIRAS, ALGARVE RIBATEJO ESTREMADURA ROSE AND SPARKLINGS.

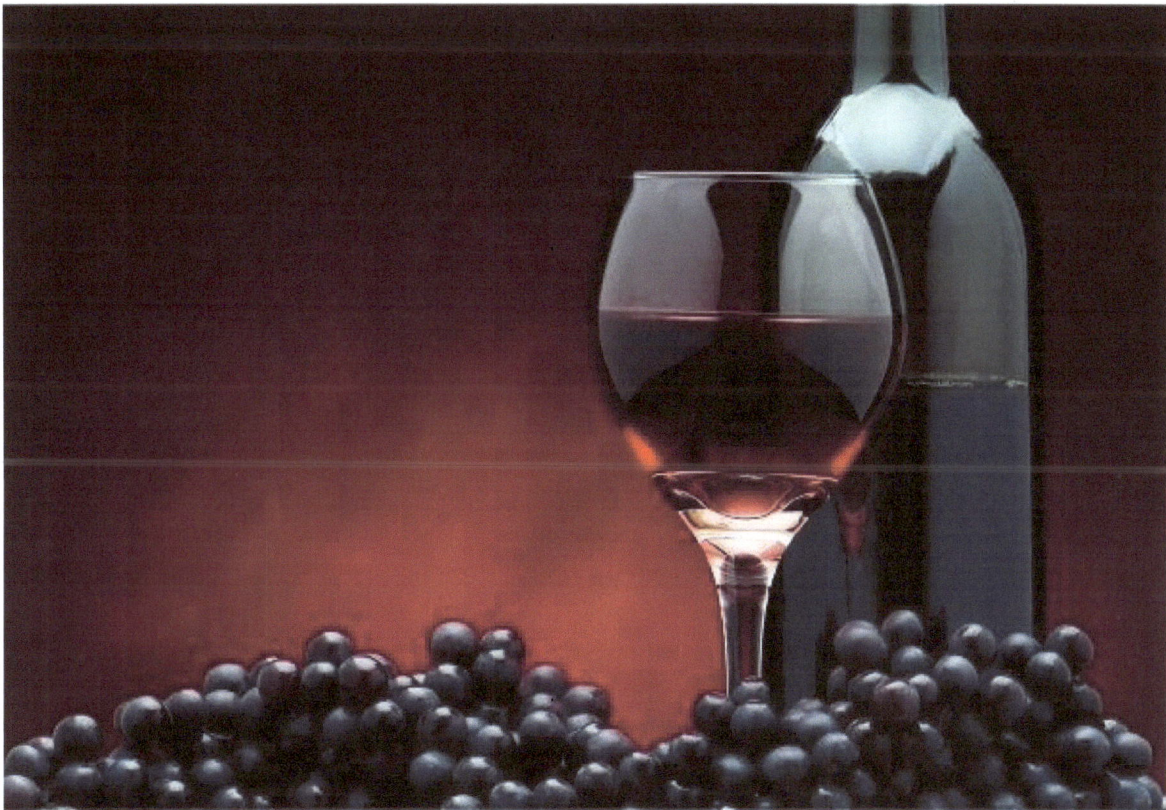

LET US SPEAK OF THE "GIN"

Native of Holland and popularized in England, the "King of Cocktails" was popularized in New York.

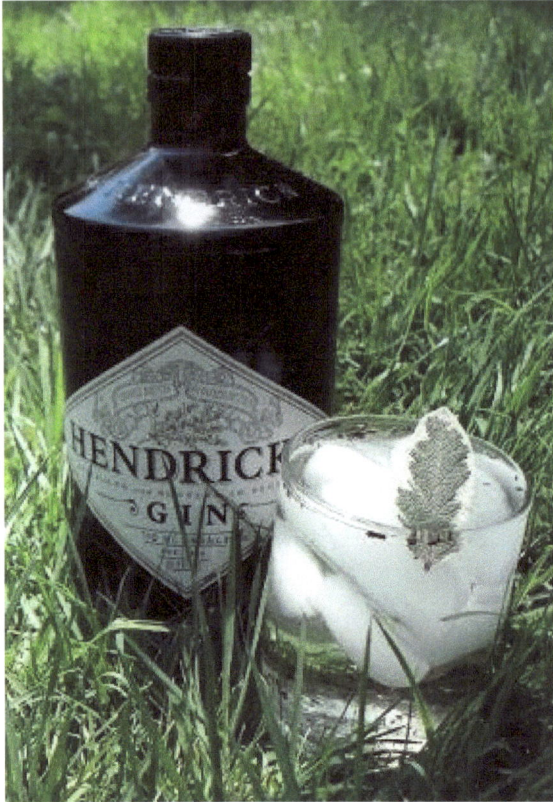

Its distillation technique, since remote times, had as a main objective to obtain spirits with medicinal and curative purposes. Man's ingenuity found alternatives coming from secondary effects of such hipocratic remedies, turning the distilled spirits into "fountains of joy", delights, eroticism, vigor and unfortunately, if consumed in excess, it can lead to negative consequences.

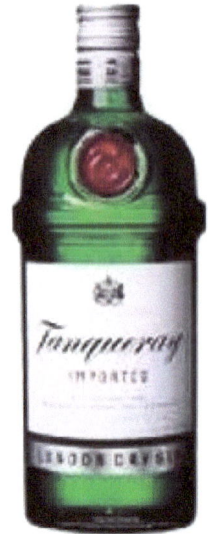

The origin of this spirit is attributed to Franciscus de la Boe (1614-72), medicine professor of the University of Leiden, Holland, who was dedicated to the spirit distillation process of barley and rye, combined with the juniper India berries (*juniperus communis)*, a copper like shrub of the cypress family. De la Boe then added certain curative and aromatic botanical ingredients, creating a medicinal remedy with diuretic properties. In a short time, the stomach and kidney ailments, and gout condition, were treated with certain success by the distilled juniper berries. This spirit, well-known by its French name, *"Genievre"*, was changed to *"Genever"* by the Dutch, who 1792 already produced 14 million gallons annually of the aforementioned "medicine" mainly produced for Export. The door was opened by the British troops during the *"Thirty Year War"* in the Netherlands. Early in the long fight, the English soldiers became fond of ingesting, in tune with its opponents a good doses of *genever*, well-known in the battlefield as the *Dutch Courage*. This is how this spirit, of an unfamiliar name, was baptized as GIN, giving rise to the beginning of a deep routed tradition in Great Britain.

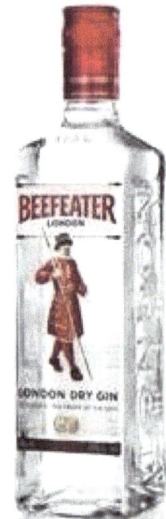

At the present time, if we take a stroll by Soho or other districts of the Old London. A signage reading "GIN" appears as a synonymous advertiser of a bar or tavern.

The Gin, name adopted in Spain when it made its appearance in the Market at the end of the Napoleonic Wars, is the first exotic spirit appearing in Europe. Gin is not a simple distilled spirit of grain like Vodka, although the technique is identical. Nevertheless, due to its original principle, the botanical and herbal ingredients, in conjunction with the producers creativity with easy access to spices originating in five continents, offer a spirit with infinite aromas.

Gin monopolized the Western Europe Market in two styles, semidry Dutch and the London Dry Gin, and undertook its trip to America, Australia, New Zealand and South Africa. The consumer, delighted with this different spirit, still demanded a formula without precedents and the producers were conscious of this deficiency. The Gin was tasted straight or with little ice. Sometimes it was mixed with seltzer and drops of lemon. Something lacked to popularize the product. **America! America!** Autumn 1912. It rained torrentially in New York. Most of the guests of the Knickerbocker Hotel went to the bars hoping the opportune moment to be able to go out into the streets. The head Bartender, Giuliano Martini, an Italian immigrant from *Arma di Taggia* stated: **"Now or never".** Addressing the clients in a loud voice, he announced the birth of unique new cocktail offered by the Hotel to calm its restless clients. "What cocktail you are referrinmg to that we already know?" Prepared and served. Seconds of silence and a unanimous loud applause.

The Martini, considered to date as the" King of the Cocktails", had been born.

Original Recipe:

1 oz. of Gin.
½ oz. French dry vermouth
2 drops Bitter Orange.
Stir with Little ice in a mixing glass.
Served in Cocktail glass.
Decorate with olive or lemon peel

It'll last forever!.

WHAT YOU MUST NOT FORGET...!

WHAT IS WINE?

This beverage, the oldest on record after water, necessary for the development of life itself, is the result of a simple organic chemical formula that sets in motion a process of fermentation. Sugar + Yeast= Alcohol CO2 + Carbon Dioxide.

Flowers, roots and the majority of fruits can be regarded as ingredients to produce certain types of fermented beverages, but our protagonist is juice extracted from ripe grapes, specifically of the European species "Vitis Vinifera" ideal for the production of wine. The grape juice provides the sugar to the formula by reacting slowly with the different wild yeasts contained in the grape skin, transforming them into alcohol and also producing carbon dioxide (CO_2), a gas that vaporizes into the atmosphere.

HIGHEST IMPORTANCE DATA

The word wine is derived from Latin, Vinum, which in turn comes from the Greek Oinos or Woinos, these being the only linguistic terms documented. The vast majority of research indicates that wine began as a mere accident. A typical anecdotal example is the old story about a family celebrating a joyous afternoon picnic in a wooded area where the vines grew wild. The grapes were an excellent fruit of great sweetness ideal to be consumed as a snack and easy to carry. The friction and pressure in the leather bags by using a primitive method of transportation, caused the crushing of the grapes, allowing the yeast of the leather to react with the sugar, by activating the formula described above. Guests put this supposed snack to the test. After a certain period of time, the guests felt the effects of the alcohol produced and apparently, it was unanimously agreed that they had discovered the "Source of Pleasure". It created what we know today as the process to make wine. Its origin is not certain, but the experts in wine science agree that it arose in the geographical areas surrounded by the Black and Caspian Seas. Fragments of fossilized vineyards were found in Persia and Egypt dating to the years 3000 to 1000 B. C., showing that the grape was wild, being subsequently cultivated. We can also verify the existence of wine in numerous scenes, murals and tomb paintings as well as in the discovery of urns and vases of the era. The first documented mentioning of wine is contained in the Old Testament of the Bible: Genesis, Book of Noah 9:20 and subsequently in the New Testament: "The Wedding in Canaan", which recounts Jesus Christ's miracle converting the water into wine.

Around the year 2000 B.C., the "Vitis Vinifera" grape opened its way through the island of Crete starting its introduction and cultivation in Europe. The first step of vinification started in Greece and eventually was extended to the European continent with the contribution of the spirit of conquest and colonization of the Roman Empire. In the XVI Century, arose the last heir: Latin America.

WHAT IS A VINEYARD?

A vineyard is the agricultural surface for planting, cultivating and harvesting of "Vitis Vinifera" species with the purpose of using its fruit, the grape, to start the process of wine production. The universal unit for measuring agricultural extension is the hectare, equivalent to 2, 471 acres. In the United States and Australia the acre is used as the unit of surface. A vineyard production volume is calculated on the number of wine boxes (1 box= 12 bottles) that are achieved per hectare, or acre of land. The vine cultivation is an intensive and detailed work. A vineyard is a garden!

CHARACTERISTICS OF A VINEYARD

The vineyard is an ensemble of perennial wooden plants with some herbaceous elements, whose roots can hold for over a hundred years. With the passage of time, the quantity of grapes produced diminishes but the quality is generally higher. However, the long life of a vineyard, in some cases, exposed to plagues, geological changes in soil and meteorological setbacks will negatively affect the resulting wine. The vineyard cycle is annual. New leaves appear in the spring and towards the end of the season, outbreaks of bundles of grapes begin. Growth takes place during the summer months in which the vines accumulate the nutrients absorbing it from the air and the soil up to the point of maturity, with the appropriate sugar content. You can see at a glance the change of grape colors. In the month of September and occasionally during the first two weeks of October, the harvest takes place. The grapes are pressed to extract the juice completing the first step in the process of wine making. When the vineyard is destined to the production of sweet wines, the grapes are not harvested until the end of October or during the month of November. This extended time frame contributes to a *fungus* concentration in the grapes, giving them a rotten look raising to the maximum the sugar content.

Wines from Sauternes (France) and German Spatlese and Auslese styles are living examples of high quality sweet white wines produced with this system of late harvest. The vines from the time they are planted should be perfectly aligned, leaving a space or corridor between them, always oriented to the cardinal points that give them maximum exposure to the sun. They need constant care during the growth period: Eradication of weeds, not using more fertilizer than necessary, maintaining regulated irrigation to preserve the altitude of the vineyard so that clusters will not touch the ground. However, the use of pesticides against parasites and *fungi* must apply in botanical crisis times.

CLIMATE

It covers not only the meteorological aspect. In viticulture, the term "climate" is related to a uniform atmospheric condition, ideal for vine cultivation and combined with an important geological factor: the ground. Many vineyards benefit from perfect climates due to the protection of atmospheric conditions of stability. However, there is also a great proliferation of isolated microclimates protecting smaller vineyards in lower wine production areas. Integrating factors benefitting the vine cultivation are: temperature, rain, solar light, wind and the proximity of topographic elevation. We can find all or most of these features around the planet, to the north and south of the Equator, between the 30 and 50 parallels of the globe, where the moderate climate reigns consistently. The green grape does better in cool climates while the red needs a warmer environment.

NEED A SPECIAL TYPE OF LAND FOR THE CULTIVATION OF THE VINE?

Yes. A deep field with good filtration and low in nutrients, protected by a suitable climate without rain during the harvest (September/October), is definitely the perfect combination. Lands having this feature are called *Terroir* in French, the term universally adopted in viticulture to define the equation climate-soil, resorting in ideal conditions for the production of wine. For the vineyard reproduction is not necessary to use seeds, but strong and healthy previous cuttings, replanted deeply to achieve firm roots. It is also advisable to graft these cuttings into roots of other already existing vineyards.

THE ANNUAL DEVELOPMENT OF THE VINEYARD

Once the harvested grapes and the soil have been cleaned up and fertilized in the winter months, the Pruning is carried out, cutting the upper part of the plant, selecting the stronger and healthier cuttings for replanting. At the same time, the resulting grape juice from the previous crop is transferred to rest in "mother vats", high volume wooden barrels already cured for many years. During the second half of February and the beginning of March, it is necessary to plough the fields. April and May are the months in which, once again, the "terroir" is cleaned and sanitized, being also the time of the year when the new wine is transferred again to new or clean oak barrels. Many wine makers build their own with new French or American oak circled with copper rings. The vine begins to develop its clusters the first week of June at a temperature from 54 to 60 degrees Fahrenheit. The higher the temperature the faster grows the foliage. The most grown cuttings are watered slightly and the structure of the vineyard is tied with wire to wooden stakes to keep them straight. July is the month of surveillance of applying the appropriate chemical elements to ensure good health for the plant. However, if the Organic Process is undertaken, chemistry must be absent entirely. In August the grapes begin to change colors understanding that the process of maturity is next. Now is the time of all malignant herb eradication arriving during the third week of September and first days of October when the harvest begins, closing the cycle that Mother Nature gave us and was perfected by Man.

THE CONSUMER

38% of the United States adult population is a wine consumer at different levels.

The Wine Institute of Napa (California) has recently presented the consumer profile system investigating 3,500 residents of the United States. This Program described the following five categories:

Household Heads: Are typically parents between the ages of 35 and 65 living in the suburbs. They enjoy drinking wine at home at least 3 days a week and enjoy eating out 2 days a week, spending an annual average of $22,000 to $34,000 by visiting Restaurants. These represent 36% of wine consumers. Their favorite wines are typically from Italy, Australia, U.S.A., Spain and Latin America of the finest brands.

Connoisseurs Adventurers: They are sophisticated expert consumers, mostly single or divorced between the ages of 28 and 45. Company Executives, hunters of good harvest years, readers of Wine Journals or Magazines belonging to high income groups, enjoying going out to Restaurants 3 days a week. Their spending average is of $35,000 to 75,000 per year, accounting for 20% of wine consumers. Drinkers of Champagne, French wine, California high brands, Gran Reserva from Spain and fine Ports.

Social Bargain Hunters: Frequent wine drinkers, always aware of pricing and promotions, making up 14% of consumers. Parents of young adolescents who like eating out and have a moderate interest in wine. Their annual consumption expense ranges from $18,000 to $25,000. They consume wines from numerous countries such as Spain, Italy, South Africa and the U.S.A., particularly California, if reasonably priced.

The Weekly: Singles between 18 to 30 years of age. They drink wine twice a week or less, visiting a Restaurant once or twice a month, spending $12,000 to $16,000 per year. Price is the most important factor for them and they usually consume low-cost Latin American and Australian wines, representing 18% of wine drinkers.

The Frugal Conservatives: Only 12% correspond to this category. They are low-income groups who rarely visit a Restaurant. Their average expenditure is $6.00 to 7.00 per bottle.

HOW TO UNLOCK THE BEST QUALITIES OF WINE

The Wine World is complex and is made up of a large variety of elements. Besides the basic rules of fermentation, bottling and aging, we discovered, in the 300 years that have passed since the appearance of the bottle in the Industry, a myriad of methods to enhance to the maximum the *bouquet* and aromas of wine. Firstly and most importantly is storing the bottle laying down flat. Secondly, maintaining an ideal temperature (53 to 60 degrees Fahrenheit) and dimmed lighting, totally free of noise and vibration. These factors are crucial in preserving optimal quality of the wine.

In 1756, Johann Riedel, from Bohemia, a designer and manufacturer of table accessories of the finest crystal and an innovator in this thriving Industry launched a line of crystal glasses created for "freeing the soul" of wines. Its premise was a minimum thickness of crystal with a slender design, allowing a slow and long breath depending on the type of wine and have the aromas and flavors directed to the more sensitive areas of the mouth. This will increase the impact on the palate. Throughout generations, the Riedel family has improved their designs currently covering all varieties of Wine. Regarding the "spirits", the firm has revolutionized all designs for their full enjoyment. The first step for wine lovers is "copeando" when accompanying their best moments in life.

SUGGESTIONS AND RECOMENDATIONS FOR CREATING A "WINE CELLAR" AT HOME AND ORDERING IN RESTAURANTS

You can start a wine cellar at home following these recommendations of wines of different varieties.

THE FINEST AND MORE POPULAR WINES
Always drink from the glass while holding the stem.

WHITES

CHAMPAGNE: Its very name brings to mind evocation of celebrations, romance and special occasions. Its composition is based on, 26% Chardonnay, 37% Pinot Noir and 37% Pinot Meunier. There are three different styles: **Non Vintage**, an expert blend of white wines from different years, **Grand Cru**, highest class of grapes planted in 17% of its *"terroir"* and **Premier Cru,** covering 44% of the total cultivation area. Ideal for "toasts" and great for accompanying all styles of "cuisine".

SAUVIGNON BLANC: A dry white wine variety from France offering distinctive aromas and flavors of citrus fruits, melon, fig and wild herbs. Also presents creamy flavors of vanilla and spices when is placed in the oak barrels. It is especially great accompanying Blue Fish, fresh Seafood, grilled Vegetables and roasted Poultry.

CHARDONNAY: This French variety produces dry and medium-dry wines with aromas and flavors of pear, apple and tropical/citrus fruits. This is the most popular of all wines, white or red, in America, having tens of thousands of acres of land for cultivation, primarily in California. The oak barrels help greatly the aging process.Magnificent with fresh fish and seafood, light snacks, smoked white meats, grilled poultry, pork tenderloin and creamy sauces.

PINOT GRIGIO: Presently the most popular Italian wine, originally proceeding from the French variety Pinot Gris. A crunchy and fresh wine with aromas and flavors of pear, apple and lemon, holding a great minerality. A great complement of seafood, poultry, white meats and *"quiche"*.

ALBARIñO: A high quality wine from Galicia (Spain) and Portugal. This variety produces creamy wines with complex flavors of peach, apricot and citrus fruits.
Is one of the highest market values in Spain and Portugal. Succulent with fresh fish and seafood.

RIESLING: The most prestigious German variety. Of slight sweetness presents floral aromas and peach, apricot, honey and pineapple flavors. Recommended with snacks, poultry, seafood, oriental dishes and, due to its sweetness, is a great companion with desserts and cheese assortments.

REDS

SAINT EMILION: The most beautiful region and largest producer of wine from Bordeaux (France). An elegant, highly concentrated wine with a full body. The vines were cultivated in Saint Emilion since the Roman Empire times. These wines carry a great fruit taste and are moderately tannic. The two large Saint Emilion regions are classified as "Grand Cru Classé" and "Premiere Grand Cru Classé", as it is recorded on the labels. We specially recommend the more sophisticated brands in the market, "Cheval Blanc", "Chateau d'Ausone" and "Chateau d'Angelus". These wines, in general, bring aromas and flavors of pure Cassis, red ripe plums, cherry and spice. The best with roasted red meats and strong cheeses.

CABERNET SAUVIGNON: The King of the red wine varieties and the most elegant. Is the grape of more importance to Bordeaux and the most appreciated in California. This intense wine offer us aromas and flavors of dark fruit, black currant, plums and raisins, smoked oak and cedar, vanilla, spices, chocolate, coffee, tobacco and wild herbs. Its style range from "easy drinking" to highly fruity. Is intense and dense with firm tannins, inviting to a long aging. It is recommended with all kind of red meat roasts and stews. Great with strong cheeses and pastas in general.

MERLOT: This wine, also from the Bordeaux area, has captured the attention of the "every day" consumer. Is refined and elegant with a great complexity, been currently the most popular in the International Market. Its aromas and flavors hit the senses with its spirit of red fruit, cherry, strawberry, raspberry, oak and cedar woods, vanilla, spices, chocolate, coffee, tobacco and wild herbs. Very similar to the Cabernet Sauvignon, but the body and tannins are lighter.

PINOT NOIR: This wine is recognized by maximum refinement and complex elegance typical of the French region of Burgundy. In United States it thrives in fresh climatic areas, such as northern California and Oregon. Its aromas and flavors evoke red fruits, cherry, strawberry, raspberry, vanilla, coffee, tobacco, spices and wild herbs. Recommended with *hors d'oeuvres*, soft cheeses, salmon, game, pork, red meats and veal.

SYRAH (France) – SHIRAZ (Australia): A variety relatively easy to cultivate It produces wines with a good body, smoothness and intensity. Coming from the Valley of the Rhone River in France, this variety is produced skillfully in the Estate of Washington (USA) and in Australia. Their aromas and flavors are based in essences of cherry, blackberry, and plum. Ideal with light appetizers, cheeses, lamb and venison.

SANGIOVESSE: Soul of the "Chianti", Variety pride of Italy. Throughout La Toscana, San Giovesse produces smooth and vivid wines with mature tannins.
Aromas and flavors of fresh red fruit stand out in these wines. Those of the highest Quality, denote complex tobacco and coffee flavors. The great Chianti supports magnificently the traditional Italian *cuisine*, particularly pastas in tomato sauce, *risottos*, and veal of all styles.

TEMPRANILLO: This variety is as important for Spain as the Cabernet Sauvignon is to France. The great red wines of La Rioja and Ribera del Duero are based on this variety. This versatile grape offers intense cherry and ripe strawberry flavors with firm tannins, which confer a great complexity to the wine. It combines with fresh fruit, roasts, stews and all cheeses wonderfully.

MALBEC: Originally a popular grape for high quality blends, it was taken from France to Argentina where it found ideal *terroir* and climate, becoming the official grape of the Country. At the present time Malbec is the most consumed red wine in the U.S.A.

Remember!

WINES "OLOROSOS" AND "GENEROSOS"

OPORTO: It is derived from the Portuguese city of the same name. For hundreds of years it has been the most popular wine world-wide for its divine sweetness and smoothness. Ideal as a "copeo" wine when enjoyed alone or with desserts, candies and confectionaries in general.

JEREZ: Know under the name "Sherry" internationally, it comes exclusively from the city of the same name in the region of Andalusia in south Spain. Two styles of production exist: The DRY version for "copeo" accompanying all types of appetizers and "tapas" and the CANDY, formidable with desserts and confections.

JOHN MARTIN

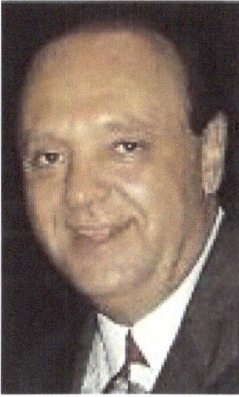

Born in Los Angeles (California) and raised in Madrid (Spain) from an early age. After finishing High School, he began his studies in the Law School of the University of Madrid with the intention of becoming a Diplomat. While studying he took a trip to Paris looking eagerly for other horizons, since the academic situation In Spain was not promising. In a short time he became fascinated with the World of the Hospitality Industry and, from Paris, he traveled to Nice and Epernay, famous for its Champagne, completing the most advanced practice of Food and Beverage within the Hotel Business and becoming Enology Licensed, topping the Wine and Spirits fields.

Subsequently, John moved to the United States with the intention of using his experience in the Food and Beverage field to join the most prestigious hotels in America such as The *Century Plaza* (Los Angeles), *Mark Hopkins* (San Francisco), *Las Vegas Hilton* (Las Vegas), *Fontainebleau* and *Doral* in Miami Beach, *Private Clubs of America* (South Florida) and High Class Restaurants that excelled due to his knowledge as Director of Operations. For the last eight years he has dedicated his professional life to consulting in the Direction of Food and Beverage.

Being a natural motivator, along with his linguistic talents, fluent in Spanish, his mother language, English, French and Italian, together with his knowledge of the Cybernetic field, made him a Natural Born Educator. Newspapers, Radio and Television frequently require his advice and for more than seventeen years worked as a Wine & Spirits Editor for the Hispanic Magazine SELECTA and, recently, joined the American CASALIFE Magazine, both considered as some of the most relevant Hispanic and Anglo Life-Style and Socio-Cultural magazines in the United States, Latin America and the Caribbean.

Contenido